THE FALLOPIAN TUBE IN INFERTILITY AND IVF PRACTICE

The Fallopian tube has until recently been a neglected structure, bypassed by in vitro fertilization (IVF) and seen only as a tube that transports the egg to the uterus. More recently, its central role as the site of fertilization and early embryogenesis has been recognized, along with the major effects of tubal disease, such as chlamydia trachomatis, on fertility. Tubal surgery is an option for those women who avoid IVF because of anxiety about medication side effects or for religious reasons. The tube is also the site for female sterilization and its reversal.

This definitive guide to the Fallopian tube and its disorders collates all these topics, with authoritative text covering the spectrum of clinically relevant topics in a digestible fashion. It will be of interest to gynecologists, specialists in reproductive medicine and infertility and family planning, and others with interest in this fascinating and underestimated organ of reproduction.

William L. Ledger, MA, DPhil, FRCOG, is Professor of Obstetrics and Gynaecology, University of Sheffield, Sheffield, UK, and Honorary Consultant in Obstetrics and Gynaecology, Jessop Wing, Royal Hallamshire Hospital, Sheffield, United Kingdom.

Seang Lin Tan, MD, MBBS, FRCOG, FRCSC, FACOG, MMed(O&G), MBA, is James Edmund Dodds Professor and Chair, Department of Obstetrics and Gynecology, McGill University, and Obstetrician and Gynecologist-in-Chief of the McGill University Health Centre, Montreal, Quebec, Canada.

Adil O. S. Bahathiq, PhD, is Associate Professor of Reproductive Endocrinology, Department of Obstetrics and Gynecology, Um-Alqura University Medical College, Mecca, Saudi Arabia.

THE FALLOPIAN TUBE IN INFERTILITY AND IVF PRACTICE

Edited by

WILLIAM L. LEDGER

University of Sheffield

SEANG LIN TAN

McGill University

ADIL O. S. BAHATHIQ

University of Um-Alqura

CAMBRIDGE
UNIVERSITY PRESS

CAMBRIDGE UNIVERSITY PRESS
Cambridge, New York, Melbourne, Madrid, Cape Town, Singapore,
São Paulo, Delhi, Dubai, Tokyo

Cambridge University Press
32 Avenue of the Americas, New York, NY 10013-2473, USA

www.cambridge.org
Information on this title: www.cambridge.org/9780521873789

First published 2010

Printed in the United States of America

A catalog record for this publication is available from the British Library.

Library of Congress Cataloging in Publication data

The fallopian tube in infertility and IVF practice / edited by William Ledger, Seang Lin Tan, Adil Bahathiq.
p. ; cm.
Includes bibliographical references and index.
ISBN 978-0-521-87378-9 (hardback)
1. Fallopian tubes – Diseases. 2. Infertility – Pathophysiology. 3. Fertilization in vitro. I. Ledger, William L. II. Tan, S. L. III. Bahathiq, Adil.
[DNLM: 1. Fallopian Tube Diseases – complications. 2. Fallopian Tube Diseases – therapy. 3. Fallopian Tubes – physiopathology. 4. Fertilization in Vitro. 5. Infertility, Female. WP 300 F1967 2010]
RG421.F363 2010
618.1′78 – dc22 2009035012

ISBN 978-0-521-87378-9 Hardback

CONTENTS

CONTRIBUTORS

Adil O. S. Bahathiq, PhD
Associate Professor of Reproductive Endocrinology, Department of Physiology, University of Um-Alqura, Mecca, Saudi Arabia

Ying C. Cheong, MD, MRCOG
Subspecialist Trainee in Reproductive Medicine and Surgery, Academic Unit of Reproductive and Developmental Medicine, University of Sheffield, Sheffield, United Kingdom

Ovrang Djahanbakhch, FRCOG, MD
Professor of Reproductive Medicine, Barts and the London School of Medicine and Dentistry, London, United Kingdom

Adrian R. Eley, PhD, MRCPath, FRCPath
Professor of Bacteriology, Department of Medical Microbiology, United Arab Emirates University, Al Ain, United Arab Emirates

Mohammad Ezzati, MD
Research Fellow, Barts and the London School of Medicine and Dentistry, London, United Kingdom

Nadia Kabli, MD
Fellow of Reproductive Endocrinology and Infertility, Department of Obstetrics and Gynecology, McGill University, Montreal, Quebec, Canada

Stephen R. Killick, MD, FRCOG, FFFP
Professor of Reproductive Medicine and Surgery, University of Hull and Hull York Medical School, Hull, United Kingdom

Hany Lashen, MB, BCh, MRCOG, MD
Clinical Senior Lecturer, Academic Unit of Reproductive and Developmental Medicine, University of Sheffield, Sheffield, United Kingdom

William L. Ledger, MA
Professor of Obstetrics and Gynaecology, Academic Unit of Reproductive and Developmental Medicine, University of Sheffield, Sheffield, United Kingdom

Kai-Fai Lee, PhD
Associate Professor, Department of Obstetrics and Gynaecology, University of Hong Kong, Queen Mary Hospital, Pokfulam, Hong Kong, China

Yin-Lau Lee, PhD
Postdoctoral Fellow, Department of Obstetrics and Gynaecology, University of Hong Kong, Queen Mary Hospital, Pokfulam, Hong Kong, China

Tin-Chiu Li, MD, PhD, MRCP, FRCOG
Professor of Obstetrics and Gynaecology, Academic Unit of Reproductive and Developmental Medicine, University of Sheffield, Sheffield, United Kingdom

Myvanwy McIlveen, B. Med (Hons), MMed, FRANZCOG, CREI
Visiting Medical Officer, Sydney IVF Newcastle and John Hunter Hospital, Newcastle, Australia

Chun Y. Ng, MBBS, MRCOG
Specialist Registrar in Obstetrics and Gynaecology, Hammersmith Hospital London, London, United Kingdom

Bassem Refaat, PhD
Academic Unit of Reproductive and Developmental Medicine, University of Sheffield, Sheffield, United Kingdom

Ertan Saridogan, PhD, FRCOG
Consultant in Gynaecology, Reproductive Medicine and Minimal Access Surgery, University College London Hospitals, Institute for Women's Health, London, United Kingdom

Seang Lin Tan, MD, MBBS, FRCOG, FRCSC, FACOG, MMed(O&G), MBA
James Edmund Dodds Professor and Chair, Department of Obstetrics and Gynecology, McGill University, Montreal, Quebec, Canada

Geoffrey H. Trew, MRCOG
Consultant in Reproductive Medicine and Surgery, Hammersmith Hospital, London, United Kingdom

Togas Tulandi, MD, MHCM
Professor of Obstetrics and Gynecology, Milton Leong Chair in Reproductive Medicine, Department of Obstetrics and Gynecology, McGill University, Montreal, Quebec, Canada

William S. B. Yeung, PhD
Professor of Obstetrics and Gynaecology, Department of Obstetrics and Gynaecology, University of Hong Kong, Queen Mary Hospital, Pokfulam, Hong Kong, China

THE FALLOPIAN TUBE IN INFERTILITY AND IVF PRACTICE

I

HISTORICAL BACKGROUND AND FUNCTIONAL ANATOMY

Adil O. S. Bahathiq and William L. Ledger

HUMAN REPRODUCTIVE TRACT

Introduction

Fetal sexual differentiation is a complicated series of events, actively programmed at the appropriate critical periods of fetal life (Table 1.1). Sex chromosomes promote the development and differentiation of the primary gonad, but the actual influences are the presence or absence of testosterone and anti-Müllerian hormone production by the testis. Brain and hypothalamic sexual identities are mainly acquired during postnatal life. Testicular Müllerian-inhibiting substance secretion causes degeneration of the Müllerian ducts. In the absence of these hormones, a female phenotype develops regardless of whether an ovary is present. The development of a female phenotype involves degeneration of the Wolffian (male) duct system, retention of the Müllerian duct system, and differentiation of female-like external genitalia.

Gonadal Differentiation

The gonad arises as an identical primordium in all embryos, poised in a precarious balance between male and female developmental pathways. Depending on whether or not a Y chromosome is present, this primordium follows a testis or ovarian fate. In vertebrates, the gonads arise as paired structures within the intermediate mesoderm, which lies on either side of the embryo, filling much of the coelomic cavity between the limb buds during the first half of development. Within this region, three segments comprising the urogenital ridge are distinguished from anterior to posterior: (1) the pronephros, which includes the adrenal primordium near its caudal end; (2) the mesonephros, the central region from which the gonad arises; and (3) the metanephros, the most posterior region in which the kidney forms.[1]

Development of the Female Reproductive Tract

Müllerian ducts appear in the human embryo at 6 weeks of gestation. In the female embryo, Müllerian ducts differentiate into Fallopian tubes, the uterus, and the upper part of the vagina. In the male fetus, Müllerian ducts begin to regress at the 8th week of gestation and have disappeared by the 9th week. This regression is because of the presence of the anti-Müllerian hormone (AMH). The Müllerian duct is sensitive to AMH during a limited period of fetal development (up to

Table 1.1 Fetal Age in Weeks After the Last Menstrual Period[2]

Fetal Age (Weeks)	*Sex-differentiating Events*
	Inactivation of one X chromosome.
4	Development of Wolffian ducts.
5	Migration of primordial germ cells in the undifferentiated gonad.
6	Development of Müllerian ducts.
7	Differentiation of seminiferous tubules.
8	Regression of Müllerian ducts in male fetus.
8	Appearance of Leydig cells. First synthesis of testosterone.
9	Total regression of Müllerian ducts. Loss of sensitivity of Müllerian ducts in the female fetus.
9	First meiotic prophase in oogonia.
10	Beginning of masculinization of external genitalia.
10	Beginning of regression of Wolffian ducts in the female fetus.
12	Fetal testis is in the internal inguinal ring.
12–14	Male penile urethra is completed.
14	Appearance of first spermatogonia.
16	Appearance of first ovarian follicles.
17	Numerous Leydig cells. Peak of testosterone secretion.
20	Regression of Leydig cells. Diminished testosterone secretion.
24	First multilayered ovarian follicles. Canalization of the vagina.
28	Cessation of oogonia multiplication.
28	Descent of testis.

8 weeks in the human fetus). The mesonephric ducts require testosterone for their development; therefore, in the female they rapidly disappear. The Fallopian tubes develop from the cranial parts of the paramesonephric ducts.[5]

DEVELOPMENT OF THE FALLOPIAN TUBE

Embryology

Between the 5th and 6th week after oocyte fertilization, a longitudinal groove called Müller's groove arises from the coelomic epithelium on each side lateral to the mesonephric duct. The edges of this groove fuse to form a canal called the Müllerian or paramesonephric duct. The Fallopian tubes develop from the cranial parts of the paramesonephric ducts, with their cranial ends remaining open and connecting the duct with the coelomic (peritoneal) cavity and the caudal end communicating with the uterine cornua. Congenital anomalies of the tube include aplasia, in which the tube fails to form; hypoplasia, in which the tube is long, narrow, and tortuous; accessory ostia; and congenital diverticula.[3,4,5]

Anatomy

The Fallopian tubes are paired, tubular, seromuscular organs whose course runs medially from the cornua of the uterus toward the ovary laterally. The tubes are situated in the upper margins of the broad ligaments between the round and utero-ovarian ligaments (Fig. 1.1). Each tube is about 10 cm long with variations

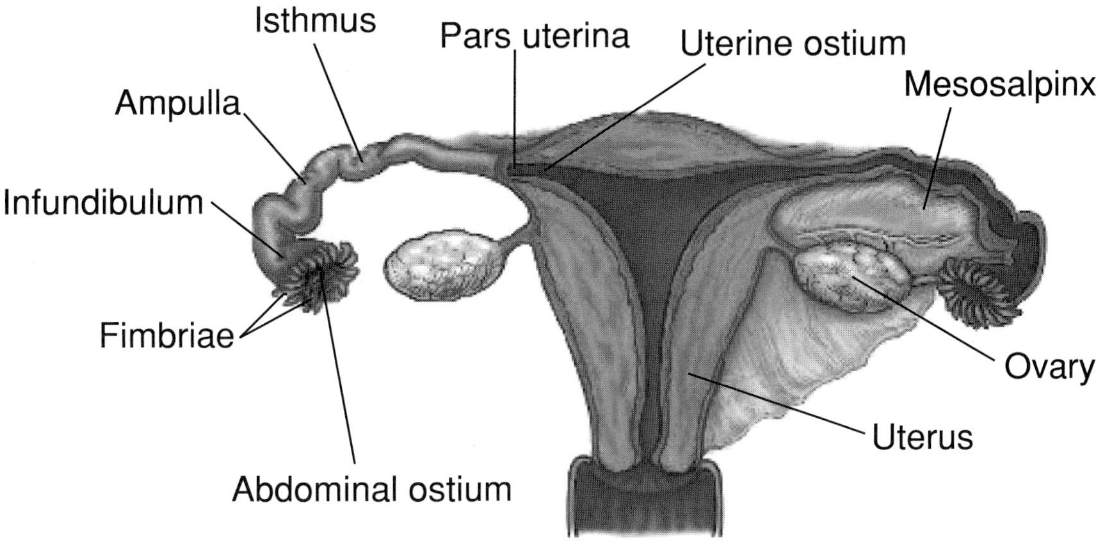

Fig. 1.1: Anatomy of the Fallopian tubes. (See Color Plate 1.)

in length from 7 to 14 cm. The abdominal ostium is situated at the base of a funnel-shaped expansion of the tube, the infundibulum, the circumference of which is enhanced by irregular processes called fimbriae. The ovarian fimbria is longer and more deeply grooved than the others and is closely applied to the tubal pole of the ovary. Passing medially, the infundibulum opens into the thin-walled ampulla, which forms more than half the length of the tube and is 1 or 2 cm in outer diameter. The isthmus is a round and cordlike structure constituting the medial one-third of the tube and 0.5–1 cm in outer diameter. The interstitial or conual portion of the tube continues from the isthmus through the uterine wall to empty into the uterine cavity.

Structure of the Fallopian Tube

The Fallopian tube or uterine tubes (Fig. 1.2) are derived from the Müllerian ducts and are paired, tubular, seromuscular organs attached laterally to the ovary and medially to the uterus fundus. They are about 7–14 cm long and are covered by peritoneum, which duplicates to form one of its loose attachments (the mesosalpinx) to the broad ligament. Their narrow proximal portion, the isthmus, begins at the uterotubal junction and extends distally to the ampulla. It is 2–3 cm long with a narrow lumen ranging from 0.1–1.0 mm in diameter.[6] The isthmic mucosa is arranged into four primary mucosal folds, with fewer ciliated cells than the other regions of the tube.

The next part is the ampullary part, which has an expanding lumen and a convoluted endosalpingeal mucosa. The ampulla is the longest portion of the human tube, ranging from 5–8 cm in length.[6] The luminal diameter varies from 1–2 mm at its junction with the isthmus to a maximum of about 1 cm near its

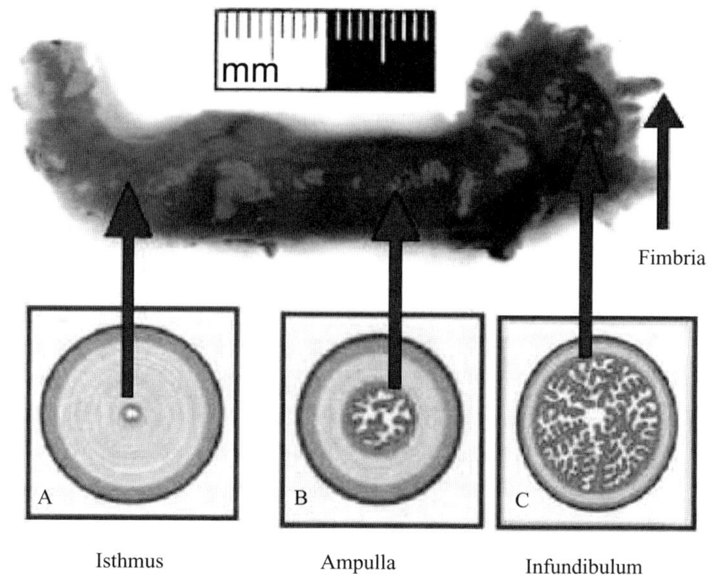

Fig. 1.2: Diagram of Fallopian tube showing different parts in cross-section: the proximal region (a) isthmus, the middle region (b) ampulla and the distal region, and (c) infundibulum. (See Color Plate 2.)

distal end. The myosalpinx in the ampulla is not organized into clear-cut muscular layers.[7] The mucosa is abundant in ciliated cells.

The distal part, the infundibulum, is the part of the tube ending in the fimbria, which is found close to the ovary. The ovarian fimbria is longer and more deeply grooved than the others and is closely applied to the tubal pole of the ovary.

The blood supply of the uterine tube comes from the vascular arch of the ovarian and uterine arteries, from which branches pass through the mesosalpinx to reach the muscular wall.

Histological Organization

The tubal wall consists of three layers: the internal mucosa (endosalpinx), the intermediate muscular layer (myosalpinx), and the outer serosa, which is continuous with the peritoneum of the broad ligament and uterus, the upper margin of which is the mesosalpinx. The endosalpinx is thrown into longitudinal folds called primary folds, which increase in number toward the fimbria and are lined by columnar epithelium of three types: ciliated, secretory, and peg cells. In the ampullary and infundibular regions, secondary folds of the tubal mucosa also exist, markedly increasing the surface areas of these segments of the tube. The myosalpinx actually consists of an inner circular and an outer longitudinal layer to which a third layer is added in the interstitial portion of the tube.[8]

Cell Form and Function of the Tubal Mucosa

The entire tubal mucosa has a columnar epithelial lining resting on connective tissue. The epithelium has two different cell types: ciliated and secretory cells. Ciliated cells are relatively square in profile, and the cilia are about 7 μm long.[6]

The percentage of ciliated cells dramatically increases from the isthmus to the fimbria.[9–11] The ciliated cells are most common in the fimbriated infundibulum. They carry upright cilia, and their primary role is to mobilize the gametes and embryo within the tube. The beat rate of the cilia is directed by the levels of estrogen and progesterone, with highest levels of activity at the time of ovulation.

The secretory cells are most abundant in the ampullary region. Secretory cells contain a granular cytoplasm characterized by fine granules, with the endoplasmic reticulum spread out irregularly.[6] In the follicular phase, the nucleus is elongated and placed with its long axis parallel to the long axis of the cell; later on in this stage the nucleus becomes more rounded in the apical of the cells.[8] These cells have several varieties of microvilli and contain high amounts of endoplasmic reticulum. Secretory material is accumulated in these cells and then released into the lumen for nourishment of the oocyte and embryo, with a possible role in the process of fertilization.

The Uterine Tube Cycle

The first description of a distinct cyclicity in the histologial appearance of the tubal epithelium in women was by Novak and Everett in 1928. They recorded that the ciliated and secretory cells underwent cyclical changes under the effect of estrogen-progesterone during the menstrual cycle. The epithelial cells reached their maximum height and degree of ciliation during the late follicular phase in the ampulla and fimbria. In the late luteal phase, atrophy and deciliation occurred, especially in the fimbrial region. Hypertrophy and reciliation started in the early follicular phase. During pregnancy and throughout the postpartum period, further atrophy and deciliation occurred.[8]

Tubal Motility

Peristaltic contraction of the smooth muscle fibers in the tubal wall allows the gametes (the sperm and egg) to be brought together, thus allowing fertilization and subsequent transport of the fertilized ovum from the normal site of fertilization in the ampulla to the normal site of implantation in the uterus. This movement is primarily regulated by three intrinsic systems: the estrogen-progesterone hormonal milieu, the adrenergic-nonadrenergic system, and prostaglandins.

Estrogens acting via their nuclear receptor stimulate tubal motility, whereas progesterone inhibits tubal motility. Before ovulation, contractions are gentle, with some individual variations in rate and pattern. At ovulation, tubal contractions become vigorous, and the mesosalpinx contracts to bring the tube in more contact with the ovary, while the fimbria contracts rhythmically to sweep over the ovarian surface. As the progesterone level rises 4–6 days after ovulation, tubal motility slows. This may lead to relaxation of the tubal musculature to allow passage of the ovum into the uterus by the action of the tubal cilia. The effects of estrogen and progesterone on oviductal motility and morphology are mediated through these steroids' receptors. The changes in receptor levels are critical in determining the functional state of the Fallopian tube.

Adrenergic innervation is thought to be involved in regulations of tubal motility, particularly isthmic motility changes. During menstruation and the proliferative (preovulatory) phase, the human tube is very sensitive to α-adrenergic compounds such as norepinephrine. After ovulation and during the luteal phase, the response to norepinephrine is decreased and the inhibitory effect of β-adrenergic compounds is more evident. Activation of the receptors by raised progesterone levels in the luteal phase leads to relaxation of the circular muscles; thus, the isthmic luminal diameter is increased and trans-isthmic passage of the fertilized ovum is facilitated.[12]

Although there is some controversy regarding the role of prostaglandins in the regulation of spontaneous tubal motility, it is generally accepted that prostaglandin F_{2a} (PGF_{2a}) stimulates, whereas PGE_1 and PGE_2 inhibit Fallopian tube contractions. Contrary to their differential activity on tubal motility, all three natural prostaglandins (PGF_{2a}, PGE_1, and PGE_2) stimulate ciliary activity in vitro.[13,14]

In summary, the initial rise in progesterone after ovulation causes contractions of the two inner layers of the uterotubal junction (UTJ), thus causing tubal locking of the ovum. After a few days, sensitivity of the muscles to adrenergic stimulation diminishes, whereas other factors, such as prostaglandins, dominate, leading to relaxation of the uterotubal junction and release of the fertilized ovum into the uterine cavity.

REFERENCES

1. Capel B, Swain A, Nicolis S, Hacker A, Walter M, Koopman P, et al. Circular transcripts of the testis-determining gene Sry in adult mouse testis. *Cell.* 1993;**73**:1019–30.
2. Sizonenko PC. Human sexual differentiation. In: Bertrand J, Rappaport R, and Sizonenko PC, editors. *Pediatric endocrinology.* Baltimore: Williams and Wilkins; 1993. pp. 88–99.
3. Peters H. Intrauterine gonadal development. *Fertil Steril.* 1976;**27**:493–500.
4. Acien P. Embryological observation on the female genital tract. *Hum Reprod.* 1992;**7**:437–45.
5. Robboy SJ, Taguchi O, Cunha GR. Normal development of the human female reproductive tract and alterations resulting from experimental exposure to diethylstilbestrol. *Hum Pathol.* 1982;**13**:190–8.
6. Pauerstein CJ, Eddy CA. Morphology of the fallopian tube. In: Beller FK, Schumacher GFB, eds. *The biology of the fluids of the female genital tract.* North Holland: Elsevier; 1979. pp. 299–317.
7. Vizza E, Correr S, Muglia U, Marchiolli F, Motta PM. The three-dimensional organization of the smooth musculature in the ampulla of the human fallopian tube: a new morpho-functional model. *Hum Reprod.* 1995;**10**(9):2400–5.
8. Verhage HG, Bareither ML, Jaffe RC, Akbar M. Cyclic changes in ciliation and cell height of the oviductal epithelium in women. *Am J Anat.* 1979;**156**:505–52.
9. Patek E, Nilsson L, Johannisson E. Scanning electron microscopy study of the human fallopian tube. Report I. The proliferative and secretory stages. *Fertil Steril.* 1972;**23**: 459–65.

10. Fredericks CM. Morphological and functional aspects of the oviductal epithelium. In: Siegler AM, editor. *The Fallopian tube: basic studies and clinical contributions.* New York: Futura Publishing Company Inc; 1986. pp. 67–80.
11. Crow J, Amso NN, Lewin J, Shaw RW. Morphology and ultrastructure of Fallopian tube epithelium at different stages of the menstrual cycle and menopause. *Hum Reprod.* 1994;**9**:2224–33.
12. Novak E, Everett HS. Cyclical and other variations in the tubal epithelium. *Am J Obstet Gynecol.* 1928;**16**:499–530.
13. Punnonen R, Lukola A. Binding of estrogen and progestin in the human Fallopian tube. *Fertil Steril.* 1981;**36**:610–14.
14. Press MF, Udove JA, Greene GL. Progesterone receptor distribution in the human endometrium. Analysis using monoclonal antibodies to the human progesterone receptor. *Am J Pathol.* 1988;**131**:112–24.

II

COCULTURE AND ASSISTED REPRODUCTION

William S. B. Yeung, Yin-Lau Lee, and Kai-Fai Lee

INTRODUCTION

Coculture in assisted reproduction refers to the culture of embryos with somatic cells that aim to enhance the development of the cocultured embryos. In the early 1990s, human embryo culture medium consisted essentially of inorganic salt; nutrient components such as glucose, pyruvate, and lactate; and serum albumin or serum. These culture media were suboptimal for embryo development in vitro as indicated by the low blastulation rate and implantation rate in assisted reproduction treatment. Hence, coculture was used to improve the embryo culture environment based on the assumption that the somatic cells would produce growth factors promoting the development of the embryo in culture. The use of coculture in assisted reproduction declined after the development of sequential culture,[1] which has rapidly become the method of choice for culturing human embryos because of the simplicity in the use of the sequential culture system. This chapter discusses the role of coculture in modern-day assisted reproduction. Emphasis will be on coculture using oviductal cells, which is the theme of this book.

OVIDUCT AND EARLY EMBRYO DEVELOPMENT

The oviduct has long been thought to be a passive conduit for the passage of the gamete and embryo in the early reproductive events. Although direct evidence is lacking, there are three lines of circumstantial evidence (mainly from animal studies) that indicate the oviduct has an additional function in enhancing the development of preimplantation embryos. The first line of evidence comes from observations of the cyclical changes in the development and activity of the ciliated cells and secretory cells of primate oviduct in the reproductive cycle. The second line of evidence derives from reports showing expression of growth factors in the oviduct and the corresponding receptors in the preimplantation embryo or vice versa. In addition, some of the oviductal growth factors are expressed in a cyclical manner. The third line of evidence includes studies reporting embryotrophic activity of oviductal cell coculture and growth factors that are found to be expressed in the oviduct. These observations highlight the possible biochemical communication between the oviductal cells and the embryos in regulating preimplantation embryo development.

COCULTURE IN ASSISTED REPRODUCTION

Oviductal Coculture in Clinical-Assisted Reproduction

The oviduct is the natural site of early embryo development. The period when we culture the embryos in assisted reproduction is mainly the time when they should be in the oviduct in vivo. Based on the belief that the oviduct should provide the best microenvironment for embryo development, several groups used oviductal cells as the helper cells for coculture in assisted reproduction. In experimental condition, oviductal cells decrease embryo fragmentation,[2] increase the rate of blastulation,[2,3] hatching,[4] and the number of cells per blastocyst[3] of human embryos.

Clinical studies including prospective randomized trials using oviductal cell coculture[5–12] had been reported. All except one[10] demonstrated either an improvement in embryo quality or pregnancy/implantation rate after coculture with oviductal cells of human or animal origin. The indications for coculture were advanced age,[9] multiple implantation failures in assisted reproduction,[6,9] and high basal follicle-stimulating hormone (FSH) level,[13] whereas coculture was inefficient in patients with good prognosis, such as young age (<age 35) and attending the first assisted reproduction cycle.[7]

Despite the positive findings on oviductal cell coculture, it is not used in assisted reproduction programs because of the extra resources required for its implementation. These resources include additional incubators, cryopreservation facilities, and manpower for the culture and storage of the donated oviductal cells and the need for screening of donors for infectious disease. Moreover, the donors of oviduct are limited. The use of oviduct of animal origin is not advisable because of the risk of transferring unknown disease from the donor animals to the human.

Coculture Studies with Other Somatic Cells in Clinical IVF

Cells other than oviductal cells, including granulosa cells, Vero cells, and endometrial cells, have been used for coculture. Currently, only homologous endometrial cell coculture is still practicing in assisted reproduction.[14,15] This is because an endometrial sample is easy to obtain from the patient for her own use, thus eliminating the need for screening donated endometrial samples for infectious disease. Endometrial cells are also easy to grow in culture. Besides, blastocyst encounters the endometrial cells in vivo providing a physiological basis for the use of these cells.

Efficacy of Coculture

The efficacy of coculture varies with the helper cells used. Although different helper cells can stimulate development of embryos in coculture, oviductal epithelial cells seem to provide a better support to the cocultured embryos, consistent with the assumption that the in vivo oviductal microenvironment is best for preimplantation embryo development. Oviductal epithelial cells are better than granulosa cells,[16] oviductal stromal cells or endometrial epithelial cells,[17] and fetal uterine fibroblast[7] in producing high-quality bovine embryos. The posttransfer development of sheep embryos after oviductal coculture is superior to those after fibroblast coculture, although both cell types stimulate embryo development in culture.[18] Human Fallopian tube epithelial cells are more efficient than oviductal fibroblasts in supporting mouse embryo development.[19] Human fibroblasts did not enhance the success rate of assisted reproduction when compared to medium alone culture in a prospectively randomized study.[20] The differential efficacy of the various helper or supporting cells in enhancing embryo development is probably because of their varied ability in the production of embryotrophic factors such as growth factors. For instance, human Fallopian tube cells but not buffalo rat liver cells express leukemia inhibitory factor (LIF) and interleukin-6 (IL-6) and possibly also activins.[21]

COCULTURE AND SEQUENTIAL CULTURE

Sequential culture refers to the use of more than one media for culturing embryos at different stages of development. Usually two media are used; one for the precompaction stages and the other for the postcompaction stages. The rationale of sequential culture is based on the knowledge of the changing metabolic needs of preimplantation embryos before and after compaction. This culture method is currently the method of choice for culturing embryos to the blastocyst stage in most assisted reproduction programs, because it requires minimal additional resources that most assisted reproduction centers can afford and it also does not have the limitations associated with coculture mentioned earlier.

The culture condition in sequential culture is not yet fully optimal because the development of embryos in such a system can still be improved under certain conditions. The development of human embryo in sequential culture systems is enhanced when the media are supplemented with granulocyte-macrophage colony-stimulating factor (GM-CSF)[22] and insulin-like growth factor-1 (IGF-1).[23] Human Fallopian tube cell coculture in sequential culture medium also improves the hatching rate of mouse embryos when compared to sequential culture alone.[24] The latter study suggests that oviductal cell coculture and sequential culture are not mutually exclusive.

It would be ideal if one can have the oviductal embryotrophic activity in the sequential culture system without the use of oviductal cells. This can be accomplished provided that the components and their composition in the oviductal microenvironment or in the oviductal coculture system are known. These data would allow us to simulate the oviductal microenvironment in vitro and to eliminate the complication involved in the use of donor oviductal tissue.

SIMULATION OF OVIDUCTAL MICROENVIRONMENT

The idea of simulating the oviductal microenvironment to improve embryo development has been practiced for many years. Early preimplantation embryos grow in the oviductal fluid in vivo. Culture media based on the salt concentrations of oviduct, such as human tubal fluid medium and mouse oviductal fluid medium, have been used to culture human and mouse embryos, respectively. The development of mouse[25] embryos cultured in media with nutrient concentration found in the oviductal fluid is superior to those cultured in conventional media.

Apart from the salt and nutrient, researchers are also interested in the growth factor environment in the oviduct. A large number of growth factors such as IGF-1 and LIF are produced in the oviductal epithelium.[26] Although there are a number of studies on the embryotrophic effect of growth factors on the development of animal embryos, similar studies on human embryos are few because of their limited availability for research. Nevertheless, supplementation of IGF-1 and LIF to the culture medium improves human embryo development; LIF enhances blastulation,[27] while IGF-1 reduces apoptosis[28] and increases the number of cells in the inner cell mass[23] of human embryos.

One of the most well-characterized embryotrophic growth factors is GM-CSF. It is expressed in the oviduct of the mouse,[29] sheep,[30] cow,[31] and human.[32] Its expression in human peaks in the preimplantation period.[32] Supplementation of GM-CSF to culture medium stimulates preimplantation embryo development of sheep,[30] mouse,[33] and human.[22] In mouse, GM-CSF treatment induces glucose uptake, enhances proliferation of the inner cell mass cells, blastulation, hatching and implantation of the treated embryos,[33,34] increases viable progeny, and improves postnatal growth after embryo transfer.[34] Mice deficient in GM-CSF have reduced fertility with impairment in fetal growth and viability.[35] Human embryos treated with GM-CSF have higher blastulation and hatching rates, and more cells in the inner cell mass and trophectoderm of blastocysts.[35] The stimulatory effect of GM-CSF on human embryos acts through a novel receptor mechanism that reduces apoptosis in the inner cell mass.[36] Two recent studies suggest that GM-CSF could be important when the preimplantation embryos are under stress, such as in medium deprived of protein[37] and after the freeze-thaw process.[38]

Data are emerging that the preimplantation embryos modulate gene expression of the oviduct. For instance, cultured human Fallopian tube cells produce more IGF-1 binding protein-3 in the presence of embryos.[39] Mouse 8-cell embryos and morula express high levels of transforming growth factor β-1 (TGFβ-1) mRNA, but they do not produce functional receptor of TGFβ-1 until the blastocyst stage,[40] suggesting that TGFβ-1 from early embryos is for paracrine rather than autocrine regulation. On the other hand, TGFβ-1 receptor is expressed in the oviduct throughout the preimplantation period,[40] consistent with a paracrine action of TGFβ-1 between the early embryos and the oviduct.

In order to confirm the modulatory action of embryos on oviductal gene expression, mouse experiments had been performed such that preimplantation embryos were transferred to one oviduct and oocytes were transferred to the contralateral oviduct. Comparison of the gene expression by subtractive suppression hybridization confirmed differential expression of genes in the two oviducts,[41] and that the expression of a panel of genes such as phospholipid transfer protein is induced in the presence of embryos.[42] Among the upregulated genes, demilune cell parotid protein enhances mouse preimplantation embryo development,[43] indicating that the embryos can stimulate the oviduct to produce embryotrophic factors. More research is necessary to identify and study the role of oviductal embryotrophic factors induced by the preimplantation embryos.

SIMULATION OF OVIDUCTAL COCULTURE ENVIRONMENT WITHOUT OVIDUCTAL CELLS

Oviductal coculture improves embryo development. Should the mechanisms of coculture embryotrophic effect be known, it would be possible to simulate the coculture environment without using the oviductal cells. Studies are being conducted along this line. There are two main proposed mechanisms for the oviductal coculture effect. They are *positive conditioning* and *negative conditioning*, which refers to the production of embryotrophic factors and the removal of suboptimal culture condition respectively by the oviductal cells. Negative conditioning is likely to be an artifact in culture because of the insufficiency in the current culture condition. Thus the helper cells help the development of cocultured embryos by reducing the level of superoxide or by adjusting the nutrient concentration in the culture medium.[26]

Knowledge of the positive conditioning mechanism has direct implication on embryo culture because of its potential in reproducing the coculture effects simply by supplementing the culture medium with embryotrophic components from the oviduct. Human Fallopian tube cells express epidermal growth factor, colony-stimulating factor-1, LIF, and IL-6.[21] The embryotrophic factors accumulate in the culture medium during culture.[26] In addition, human Fallopian tube expresses activin and follistatin as putative growth factors. Apart from growth factors, other molecules or partially purified fractions, some with unknown identities, also serve as embryotrophic factors. Three fractions that stimulate mouse embryo development from the spent medium after human Fallopian tube cells culture had been isolated.[44] These fractions named embryotrophic factor-1 (ETF-1), ETF-2, and ETF-3 have molecular size >100-kDa, which is much larger than commonly known growth factors. They have differential spatial and temporal activities on mouse embryo development.[45] ETF-1 and ETF-2 are more potent in the first 2 days of culture after fertilization. They increase the cell number in the inner cell mass of the treated embryos. On the other hand, ETF-3 is active from around compaction. It promotes the development of the trophectoderm, which in turns leads to the production of larger blastocysts that hatched, attached to, and spread on the culture dish more efficiently than the untreated control.

Data are available suggesting that human Fallopian tube cells affect several processes in embryo development. Human Fallopian tube cell coculture enhances proliferation and reduces apoptosis in mouse morula and blastocyst[46] by suppressing caspases activities and by maintaining mitochondrial function.[47] There are differential expression of genes between the cocultured embryos and those cultured in medium alone.[48] ETF-3 treatment reproduces some of these biological effects seen in coculture. It enhances proliferation and suppresses apoptosis of mouse embryos.[49] These are likely to act through multiple pathways as it affects the expression of a panel of genes in the treated embryos.[50] Its ability to produce blastocysts of larger size is probably related to its stimulatory activity on the expression of β1 subunit of sodium-potassium adenosine triphosphatase,[49] which affects the formation of the blastocoel.

One main obstacle in the identification of oviductal embryotrophic factors is that the donated oviductal cells do not produce sufficient amount of embryotrophic factors for characterization, and that the oviductal cells become fibroblast-like and stop producing embryotrophic factors after prolonged culture. Therefore, an immortalized human oviductal cell line was established to solve this problem.[51] The cell line retains various characteristics of the primary oviductal cells, including expression of cytokeratin and estrogen receptor, and production of oviduct-specific glycoprotein as well as some embryotrophic factors. With the use of the immortalized oviductal cells, ETF-3 was identified as a mixture containing complement protein-3 (C3) and its derivatives.[52]

The immunoreactivity of C3 is detected in the oviductal epithelium of human and mouse. Both the mRNA and protein of C3 are also expressed in the immortalized oviductal cells but not in the Vero cells and the fibroblasts.[52] Among the derivatives of C3 tested, inactivated complement-3b (iC3b) is most potent in stimulating mouse embryo development, while C3 is not embryotrophic.[52] Embryos treated with iC3b have higher blastulation rate, hatching rate, and their blastocysts are larger in size. Our unpublished data show that the oviductal cells and the cocultured mouse embryos cooperate to produce embryotrophic iC3b, such that C3 convertase produced by the oviduct converts oviduct-derived C3 into complement-3b, which is transformed into iC3b by complement receptor 1-related gene/protein Y on the surface of the mouse embryos. This mechanism enables the embryotrophic iC3b to be formed next to the embryos and thus maximize the efficiency of the embryotrophic factor. Research is ongoing to determine the possibility of using these in clinical assisted reproduction.

CONCLUSION

Nature provides the best condition for the development of embryos, which are exposed to the oviductal microenvironment for most of the preimplantation period. Data are emerging showing that the embryos can modulate oviductal microenvironment through interaction with the oviduct. While simulation of the salt and nutrient composition in the oviduct has been used to improve the efficacy of culture medium in supporting preimplantation embryo development, these media still contain only a small subset of the components in the oviduct. Thus, the current system is not yet fully optimal. Knowledge on the oviductal microenvironment and how it is regulated is crucial to the development of better embryo culture media.

The use of oviductal coculture is practically demanding and is unsuitable for use in routine assisted reproduction. However, coculture is a good model to study the interaction between the embryos and the oviductal cells and to identify embryotrophic factors produced by the oviductal cells. The former is especially important in humans because performing similar study in vivo is ethically impossible. The latter would enable the production of chemically defined medium with coculture embryotrophic effect but without the need of using helper cells by supplementing the embryo culture medium with recombinant form of the embryotrophic factors.

It is well established that the metabolic requirement of the preimplantation embryos changes as the embryo grows. The reproductive tract responds to fit the changing needs of the embryo. Thus, the uterine fluid and oviductal fluid have different nutrient composition. It is logical to assume that the embryotrophic factor requirement of the embryos would likewise be different, and that the embryotrophic factors from the uterus are different from that of the oviduct. The endometrial coculture system will be a good model to identify specific factors important for the well-being of the later stages of preimplantation embryo development.

ACKNOWLEDGMENT

This work was supported fully by grants (HKU39/91, HKU241/95M, HKU 7333/97M, HKU7327/00M, HKU7436/03M, and HKU7411/04M) to William S. B. Yeung and Calvin K. F. Lee from the Research Grant Council, Hong Kong.

REFERENCES

1. Gardner DK, Schoolcraft WB, Wagley L, Schlenker T, Stevens J, Hesla J. A prospective randomized trial of blastocyst culture and transfer in in vitro fertilization. *Hum Reprod.* 1998;**13**:3434–40.
2. Bongso A, Ng SC, Sathananthan H, Lian NP, Rauff M, Ratnam S. Improved quality of human embryos when co-cultured with human ampullary cells. *Hum Reprod.* 1989;**4**:706–13.
3. Vlad M, Walker D, Kennedy RC. Nuclei number in human embryos co-cultured with human ampullary cells. *Hum Reprod.* 1996;**11**:1678–86.
4. Yeung WSB, Ho PC, Lau EY, Chan STH. Improved development of human embryos in vitro by a human oviductal cell co-culture system. *Hum Reprod.* 1992;**7**:1144–9.
5. Wiemer KE, Hoffman DI, Maxson WS, Eager S, Muhlberger B, Fiore I, et al. Embryonic morphology and rate of implantation of human embryos following co-culture on bovine oviductal epithelial cells. *Hum Reprod.* 1993;**8**:97–101.
6. Wiemer KE, Garrisi J, Steuerwald N, Alikani M, Reing AM, Ferrara TA, et al. Beneficial aspects of co-culture with assisted hatching when applied to multiple-failure in-vitro fertilization patients. *Hum Reprod.* 1996;**11**:2429–33.
7. Wiemer KE, Cohen J, Tucker MJ, Godke RA. The application of co-culture in assisted reproduction: 10 years of experience with human embryos. *Hum Reprod.* 1998;**13 Suppl 4**:226–38.
8. Morgan K, Wiemer K, Steuerwald N, Hoffman D, Maxson W, Godke R. Use of videocinematography to assess morphological qualities of conventionally cultured and cocultured embryos. *Hum Reprod.* 1995;**10**:2371–6.

9. Tucker MJ, Ingargiola PE, Massey JB, Morton PC, Wiemer KE, Wiker SR, et al. Assisted hatching with or without bovine oviductal epithelial cell co-culture for poor prognosis in-vitro fertilization patients. *Hum Reprod.* 1994;**9**:1528–31.
10. Tucker MJ, Morton PC, Wright G, Ingargiola PE, Sweitzer CL, Elsner CW, et al. Enhancement of outcome from intracytoplasmic sperm injection: does co-culture or assisted hatching improve implantation rates? *Hum Reprod.* 1996;**11**:2434–7.
11. Yeung WSB, Lau EY, Chan ST, Ho PC. Coculture with homologous oviductal cells improved the implantation of human embryos – a prospective randomized control trial. *J Assist Reprod Genet.* 1996;**13**:762–7.
12. Bongso A, Ng SC, Fong CY, Anandakumar C, Marshall B, Edirisinghe R, et al. Improved pregnancy rate after transfer of embryos grown in human fallopian tubal cell coculture. *Fertil Steril.* 1992;**58**:569–74.
13. Wiemer KE, Hu Y, Cuervo M, Genetis P, Leibowitz D. The combination of coculture and selective assisted hatching: results from their clinical application. *Fertil Steril.* 1994;**61**:105–10.
14. Mercader A, Garcia-Velasco JA, Escudero E, Remohí J, Pellicer A, Simón C. Clinical experience and perinatal outcome of blastocyst transfer after coculture of human embryos with human endometrial epithelial cells: a 5-year follow-up study *Fertil Steril.* 2003;**80**:1162–8.
15. Spandorfer SD, Pascal P, Parks J, Clark R, Veeck L, Davis OK, et al. Autologous endometrial coculture in patients with IVF failure: outcome of the first 1,030 cases. *J Reprod Med.* 2004;**49**:463–7.
16. Wiemer KE, Watson AJ, Polanski V, McKenna AI, Fick GH, Schultz GA. Effects of maturation and co-culture treatments on the developmental capacity of early bovine embryos. *Mol Reprod Dev.* 1991;**30**:330–8.
17. Goff AK, Smith LC. Effect of steroid treatment of endometrial cells on blastocyst development during co-culture. *Theriogenology.* 1998;**49**:1021–30.
18. Gandolfi F, Moor RM. Stimulation of early embryonic development in the sheep by co-culture with oviduct epithelial cells. *J Reprod Fertil.* 1987;**81**:23–8.
19. Liu LP, Chan STH, Ho PC, Yeung WSB. Human oviductal cells produce high molecular weight factor(s) that improves the development of mouse embryo. *Hum Reprod.* 1995;**10**:2781–6.
20. Wetzels AM, Bastiaans BA, Hendriks JC, Goverde HJ, Punt-van der Zalm AP, Verbeet JG, et al. The effects of co-culture with human fibroblasts on human embryo development in vitro and implantation. *Hum Reprod.* 1998;**13**:1325–30.
21. Barmat LI, Worrilow KC, Paynton BV. Growth factor expression by human oviduct and buffalo rat liver coculture cells. *Fertil Steril.* 1997;**67**:775–9.
22. Sjoblom C, Wikland M, Robertson SA. Granulocyte-macrophage colony-stimulating factor promotes human blastocyst development in vitro. *Hum Reprod.* 1999;**14**:3069–76.
23. Lighten AD, Moore GE, Winston RM, Hardy K. Routine addition of human insulin-like growth factor-I ligand could benefit clinical in-vitro fertilization culture. *Hum Reprod.* 1998;**13**:3144–50.
24. Xu JS, Chan STH, Lee WM, Lee KF, Yeung WSB. Differential growth, cell proliferation, and apoptosis of mouse embryo in various culture media and in coculture. *Mol Reprod Dev.* 2004;**68**:72–80.
25. Gardner DK, Leese HJ. Concentrations of nutrients in mouse oviduct fluid and their effects on embryo development and metabolism in vitro. *J Reprod Fertil.* 1990;**88**:361–8.
26. Yeung WSB, Xu JS, Lee CKF. The oviduct and preimplantation embryo development. *Reprod Med Rev.* 2002;**10**:21–44.
27. Dunglison GF, Barlow DH, Sargent IL. Leukaemia inhibitory factor significantly enhances the blastocyst formation rates of human embryos cultured in serum-free medium. *Hum Reprod.* 1996;**11**:191–6.

28. Spanos S, Becker DL, Winston RM, Hardy K. Anti-apoptotic action of insulin-like growth factor-I during human preimplantation embryo development. *Biol Reprod.* 2000;**63**:1413–20.
29. Robertson SA, Mayrhofer G, Seamark RF. Uterine epithelial cells synthesize granulocyte-macrophage colony-stimulating factor and interleukin-6 in pregnant and nonpregnant mice. *Biol Reprod.* 1992;**46**:1069–79.
30. Imakawa K, Helmer SD, Nephew KP, Meka CS, Christenson RK. A novel role for GM-CSF: enhancement of pregnancy specific interferon production, ovine trophoblast protein-1. *Endocrinol.* 1993;**132**:1869–71.
31. de Moraes AA, Paula LF, Chegini N, Hansen PJ. Localization of granulocyte-macrophage colony-stimulating factor in the bovine reproductive tract. *J Reprod Immunol.* 1999;**42**:135–45.
32. Zhao Y, Chegini N. Human Fallopian tube expresses granulocyte-macrophage colony stimulating factor (GM-CSF) and GM-CSF alpha- and beta-receptors and contain immunoreactive GM-CSF protein. *J Clin Endocrinol Metab.* 1994;**79**:662–5.
33. Robertson SA, Sjoblom C, Jasper MJ, Norman RJ, Seamark RF. Granulocyte-macrophage colony-stimulating factor promotes glucose transport and blastomere viability in murine preimplantation embryos. *Biol Reprod.* 2001;**64**:1206–15.
34. Sjoblom C, Roberts CT, Wikland M, Robertson SA. Granulocyte-macrophage colony-stimulating factor alleviates adverse consequences of embryo culture on fetal growth trajectory and placental morphogenesis. *Endocrinology.* 2005;**146**:2142–53.
35. Robertson SA, Roberts CT, Farr KL, Dunn AR, Seamark RF. Fertility impairment in granulocyte-macrophage colony-stimulating factor-deficient mice. *Biol Reprod.* 1999;**60**:251–61.
36. Sjoblom C, Wikland M, Robertson SA. Granulocyte-macrophage colony-stimulating factor (GM-CSF) acts independently of the beta common subunit of the GM-CSF receptor to prevent inner cell mass apoptosis in human embryos. *Biol Reprod.* 2002;**67**: 1817–23.
37. Karagenc L, Lane M, Gardner DK. Granulocyte-macrophage colony-stimulating factor stimulates mouse blastocyst inner cell mass development only when media lack human serum albumin. *Reprod Biomed Online.* 2005;**10**:511–18.
38. Papayannis M, Eyheremendy V, Sanjurjo C, Blaquier J, Raffo FG. Effect of granulocyte-macrophage colony stimulating factor on growth, resistance to freezing and thawing and re-expansion of murine blastocysts. *Reprod Biomed Online.* 2007;**14**:96–101.
39. Lai YM, Wang HS, Lee CL, Lee JD, Huang HY, Chang FH, et al. Insulin-like growth factor-binding proteins produced by Vero cells, human oviductal cells and human endometrial cells, and the role of insulin-like growth factor-binding protein-3 in mouse embryo co-culture systems. *Hum Reprod.* 1996;**11**:1281–6.
40. Chow JF, Lee KF, Chan STH, Yeung WSB. Quantification of transforming growth factor beta1 (TGFbeta1) mRNA expression in mouse preimplantation embryos and determination of TGFbeta receptor (type I and type II) expression in mouse embryos and reproductive tract. *Mol Hum Reprod.* 2001;**7**:1047–56.
41. Lee KF, Yao YQ, Kwok KL, Xu JS, Yeung WSB. Early developing embryos affect the gene expression patterns in the mouse oviduct. *Biochem Biophys Res Commun.* 2002;**292**: 564–70.
42. Lee KF, Kwok KL, Chung MK, Lee YL, Chow JFC, Yeung WSB. Phospholipid transfer protein (PLTP) mRNA expression is stimulated by developing embryos in the oviduct. *J Cell Biochem.* 2005;**95**:740–9.
43. Lee KF, Xu JS, Lee YL, Yeung WSB. Demilune cell parotid protein (Dcpp) from murine oviductal epithelium stimulates pre-implantation embryo development. *Endocrinol.* 2006;**147**:79–87.
44. Liu LP, Chan STH, Ho PC, Yeung WSB. Partial purification of embryotrophic factors from human oviductal cells. *Hum Reprod.* 1998;**13**:1613–19.

45. Xu JS, Cheung TM, Chan STH, Ho PC, Yeung WSB. Temporal effect of human oviductal cell and its derived embryotrophic factors on mouse embryo development. *Biol Reprod.* 2001;**65**:1481–8.
46. Xu JS, Cheung TM, Chan STH, Ho PC, Yeung WSB. Human oviductal cells reduce the incidence of apoptosis in cocultured mouse embryos. *Fertil Steril.* 2000;**74**:1215–19.
47. Xu JS, Chan STH, Ho PC, Yeung WSB. Human oviductal cells coculture maintained the mitochondrial function and decreased the caspase's activity of cleavage-staged mouse embryos. *Fertil Steril.* 2003;**80**:178–83.
48. Lee KF, Chow JF, Xu JS, Chan STH, Ip SM, Yeung WSB. A comparative study of gene expression in murine embryos developed in vivo, cultured in vitro, and cocultured with human oviductal cells using messenger ribonucleic acid differential display. *Biol Reprod.* 2001;**64**:910–17.
49. Xu JS, Lee YL, Lee KF, Kwok KL, Luk JM, Lee WM, Yeung WSB. Embryotrophic factor-3 from human oviductal cell enhances proliferation, suppresses apoptosis, and stimulates the expression of β1 subunit of sodium-potassium ATPase of mouse embryos. *Hum Reprod.* 2004;**19**:2919–26.
50. Lee YL, Lee KF, Xu JS, Kwok KL, Luk JM, Lee WM, et al. Embryotrophic factor-3 from human oviductal cells affects the messenger ribonucleic expression of mouse blastocyst. *Biol Reprod.* 2003;**68**:375–82.
51. Lee YL, Lee KF, Xu JS, Wang YL, Tsao SW, Yeung WSB. Establishment and characterization of an immortalized human oviductal cell line. *Mol Reprod Dev.* 2001;**59**:400–9.
52. Lee YL, Lee KF, Xu JS, He QY, Chiu JF, Lee WM, Luk JM, Yeung WSB. The embryotrophic activity of oviductal cell derived complement C3b and iC3b – a novel function of complement protein in reproduction. *J Biol Chem.* 2004;**279**:12763–8.

III

PHYSIOLOGY AND PATHOPHYSIOLOGY OF TUBAL TRANSPORT: CILIARY BEAT AND MUSCULAR CONTRACTILITY, RELEVANCE TO TUBAL INFERTILITY, RECENT RESEARCH, AND FUTURE DIRECTIONS

Ovrang Djahanbakhch, Mohammad Ezzati, and Ertan Saridogan

INTRODUCTION

Effective tubal transport of the gametes and embryo is essential for a successful spontaneous pregnancy. Although there is much to be discovered about the mechanisms involved, tubal transit is a far more complicated process than initially thought. With the advancement of in vitro fertilization (IVF) and its reasonable success rate, there was a widespread assumption that the physiological role of Fallopian tubes was little more than provision of a passive conduit for the sperm, oocytes, and embryos. However, there is now increasing evidence that a complex system of trilateral interactions among the tubal epithelium, tubal fluid, and tubal contents (including sperm, ova, and embryos) simultaneously plays a permissive role for a successful spontaneous pregnancy on the one hand and prevention of unwanted reproductive outcomes such as polyspermy and tubal pregnancy on the other. The mechanical component of this elusive process comprises the propulsion of gametes and embryos within the oviduct. This is achieved by complex interaction among tubal peristalsis, ciliary activity and the flow of tubal secretions.

In this chapter we aim to elaborate on the current knowledge of ciliary activity, tubal smooth muscle contractions and their physiological regulation. We also discuss the effects on ciliary function of cigarette smoking and various pathological states, including endometriosis and microbial infection, with consideration given as to how altered ciliary activity may affect fertility.

MUSCULAR CONTRACTILITY

Two distinct types of contractions have been described in the oviductal smooth muscle: sustained tonic contractions and frequent brief episodic contractions.[1–3] Sustained tonic contractions are localized to the ampullary-isthmic junction (AIJ) and the uterotubal junction (UTJ) and probably serve as a sphincter mechanism to transiently arrest the tubal transport of gametes and embryos.[4] During this transient arrest, the other type of contractions in the form of frequent but brief spells of contractions will mix the tubal passengers including the gametes and embryo with the tubal fluid. These episodic contractions are generated following the signals from multiple pacemakers that are not only scattered across the oviduct but also constantly changing location.[5] These peristaltic waves propagate in both directions for short distances at a rate of 1–2 mm per second. It is thought that the movements brought about by these contractions do not lead to any net progress in any direction.[6] Instead they might serve to increase the interactions between the gametes/embryos and the tubal secretions.[7] Receptors for ovarian steroid hormones including estradiol and progesterone have been identified in the oviductal smooth muscle cells. In-vivo concentrations of these hormones are unlikely to cause either contraction or relaxation, but it is plausible that these hormones might modulate the effects of other mediators such as noradrenaline, neuropeptide Y, vasoactive intestinal peptide (VIP), substance P, prostaglandins and nitric oxide.[8–13] Furthermore, some growth factor such as activins has been identified in the uterine tube of both human and animals, and it may be involved in the early stage of embryogenesis.[14] The cumulative effect of these agents in vivo or even in vitro is not known and therefore one should be extremely cautious with the temptation of any pharmacological intervention to optimize the tubal transport.

CILIARY MOTILITY

Although the relative significance of various mechanisms involved in tubal transport is still unclear, some studies suggest that ciliary action is the leading role in transfer of gametes and embryos. In animal studies, if muscular activity is inhibited by isoproterenol, a β-adrenergic agonist, there is no difference in total transit times through the ampulla, suggesting that the cilia alone are capable of transporting the ovum to the site of fertilization within a normal time frame.[15,16] Case reports of women with the "immotile cilia syndrome," or Kartagener's syndrome or primary ciliary dyskinesia (PCD) who were found to have no other reason for their infertility might be considered as evidence for the crucial role of cilia in tubal transport.[17–19]

Successful pregnancies that have been observed in women with this condition may be explained by a subgroup of affected individuals demonstrating some, albeit dyskinetic, ciliary action.[20–22] Ciliary dyskinesia due to various pathologies can potentially have adverse effects on the tubal transfer with subsequent impairment of the fertility. PCD is one of the conditions in which ciliary motility is impaired. Theoretically, any mutation in the genes whose products are essential for either ciliary structure or function can be responsible for the pathogenesis of this syndrome. These include defects of inner dynein arm, outer dynein arm, tubulins (α subunit and β subunit), radial spokes and other regulatory proteins whose presence and intact structure are essential for normal ciliary function.[23]

At a genetic and molecular level, considering the different mutations and subsequent structural or functional defects that can give rise to this spectrum of disease, PCD is regarded as a heterogeneous disorder. Molecular genetic studies have demonstrated multiple gene loci.[24,25] The underlying genetic and molecular defects remain unidentified in the majority of cases. However, to this point only three dynein-related genes (DNAI1, DNAH5, DNAH11) have been successfully linked to PCD.[26–28]

As the list of potential targets responsible for PCD is extremely extensive with about 250 protein and their associated genes, it is plausible that because of tissue-specific expression of axoneme-related genes, the mutations responsible for the respiratory phenotype of the PCD do not affect the ciliary function in the Fallopian tube. This might explain a handful of case reports describing normal fertility in women diagnosed with PCD.

REGULATION OF CILIARY BEAT FREQUENCY (CBF)

A variety of hormonal and neuronal stimuli influence the ciliary activity. Both calcium and adenosine triphosphate (ATP) are required for ciliary movement. In vitro studies have demonstrated that the absence of calcium in the culture medium results in cessation of ciliary motility[29] and addition of ATP increases the CBF in a dose-dependent manner.[30] Although the exact mechanism by which this might occur in vivo has not been elucidated, secretory cells have been suggested as a possible source of ATP release with a potential paracrine mode of action on the nearby ciliated cells. β-adrenergic stimulation increases ciliary activity, an effect that can be blocked by the β-adrenergic receptor blocker, propranolol, confirming the receptor specificity of this response.[31] Angiotensin II in nanomolar concentrations has been shown to stimulate CBF in vitro. This effect is inhibited by the specific type 1 angiotensin II receptor antagonist, losartan.[32] The presence of a renin–angiotensin system has been described in the human Fallopian tube, and angiotensin II receptors are present in the tubal mucosa, with immunostaining being most prominent in the proliferative phase. The role of angiotensin II in tubal function has not yet been elucidated.

It has been hypothesized that the increase in CBF after ovulation is because of rising progesterone levels in an estrogen-rich environment, which may increase the release of ATP from apically situated mitochondria within the ciliated cells, and thus increase CBF.[33] However, high-dose progesterone has been shown to inhibit CBF in vitro by up to 63 percent.[34,35] This inhibition can be reversed by the progesterone receptor antagonist and mifepristone.[34] The ovarian hormones are present in the Fallopian tube mucosa in much higher concentrations than in the general circulation because of a countercurrent exchange mechanism between the ovarian artery and the venous plexuses along the mesosalpinx.[36] Additionally, the Fallopian tube cilia are directly exposed to high levels of ovarian steroids at midcycle with the influx of follicular fluid. High levels of estrogen and progesterone in the peritoneal fluid, which is in direct communication with the tubal lumen, prolong the ciliary exposure to raised ovarian hormone levels during the secretory phase. As high concentrations of progesterone decrease CBF, the postovulatory increase in CBF may be due to alternative factors.[37,38]

Among other factors affecting the ciliary activity, animal studies in vitro have demonstrated that PGE2 (prostaglandins E_2 and F_2) and F2α both stimulate fimbrial CBF. It is believed that this effect is achieved by prostaglandin-induced release of calcium ions.[29,39] It has been suggested that either tubal mucosa or the cumulus complex around the ovum might secrete prostaglandins that stimulate ciliary activity, acting through the release of calcium ions from intracellular storage sites or the extracellular space.[33] Follicular fluid exerts a significant stimulatory effect on CBF of human Fallopian tube explants in vitro.[40] The follicular fluid of human preovulatory ovarian follicles contains high concentrations of estradiol (E2), progesterone and prostaglandins.[41–43] As part of the ovum pickup process around the time of ovulation, the fimbrial end of the Fallopian tube comes in close proximity to the dominant ovarian follicle.[44] It has been suggested that among other factors, the flow of follicular fluid into the Fallopian tube might assist in the transfer of the ovum to inside the tube.[45] Follicular fluid thus becomes the major constituent of tubal fluid immediately postovulation. It appears that prostaglandins or other factors in the follicular fluid may provide the stimulus for the increase in CBF observed in the secretory phase and that this may aid ovum pickup and transport.

OVUM TRANSPORT

Physical interaction between the fimbrial end of the tube and the ovulating follicle, in the form of a back-and-forth movement, is probably responsible for disrupting and removing the cumulus mass once the oocyte is released.[46] Although we do not have a clear picture of the mechanisms involved, it seems that the mesosalpingeal muscle plays an important role by twisting the tube and bringing the fimbria into close apposition with the ovary.[47,48] Among the possible factors influencing this process, it has been suggested that prostaglandins within follicular fluid might mediate this action by increasing the contractility of both fimbria and tubo-ovarian ligaments.[49,50]

Using transvaginal hydrolaparoscopy, Gordts et al. visualized the process of ovum retrieval. The fimbriae on the ovulatory side appeared congested and tumescent and showed pulsatile movements synchronous with the heartbeat. The cumulus mass was adherent to the fimbriae and was released from the site of rupture by the sweeping movements of the fimbriae until it disappeared between the rigid fimbrial folds.[51] There is a significant oozing of high concentrations of follicular 17ß-estradiol after ovulation. It is known that 17ß-estradiol causes an enhanced vasodilatation by stimulating endothelial nitric oxide and prostacyclin activity[52] and by decrease of protein kinase C activity.[53] This might explain the vascular changes observed in the fimbriae on the ovulation side.[51]

Ethical and technical difficulties have limited the extent to which it has been possible to study the tubal transport of ovum in women, although some experimental data have been obtained from investigations on patients undergoing salpingectomy for sterilization. Performing the operation at varying time periods following ovulation confirmed by the luteinizing hormone (LH) surge and determining the site of ovum retrieval from the tube led the researchers to conclude that the tubal transit time in humans is approximately 80 hours.[54] It takes almost 8 hours for the ovum to reach the AIJ once it is released from the follicle. Then fertilization takes place at the AIJ, and the developing embryo then appears to stay in the ampulla for 72 hours before proceeding to the UTJ.[54,55] Some researchers have suggested that increased isthmic tone around the time of ovulation, as well as the presence of a dense, tenacious mucus obliterating the isthmic lumen, might be responsible for this observed transient pause in ovum/embryo transport.[56,57] Later on, the effect of progesterone results in the disappearance of the isthmic mucus. Furthermore, downregulation of α-adrenergic receptors by inhibitory β-receptors results in the relaxation of the muscle tone. Consequently, the isthmic lumen opens and allows the transport of early embryo to the uterus.[58]

Clinical observations have suggested that a second mechanism for oocyte retrieval from the cul-de-sac or intervisceral spaces exists in the human. This secondary pickup is more likely to result in late retrieval and peritoneal transmigration of the oocyte to the oviduct on the opposite side of the ovulation. Pregnancies have been reported in women with one ovary and only a contralateral Fallopian tube. The frequency of this phenomenon has been estimated to be less than 5 percent in normal fertile women.[59] However, it is plausible that its frequency might be significantly higher in conceptions that lead to tubal implantation. The frequent association with chronic salpingitis, however, makes it difficult to attribute a relative importance score to either transmigration with possibly delayed pickup or underlying tubal pathology in the pathogenesis of tubal pregnancy.[60,61] Conversely some experimental studies have shown the possibility of oocyte retrieval by the fimbrial end of the tube from the Pouch of Douglas, because it was demonstrated that microspheres injected into the peritoneal cavity through the posterior vaginal fornix can be captured by the fimbria.[62]

PATHOPHYSIOLOGY OF TUBAL TRANSPORT

Aberrant tubal transport is implicated in numerous pathological conditions including infectious and inflammatory causes, endometriosis and smoking.

ENDOMETRIOSIS

The peritoneal microenvironment in women with endometriosis differs from normal fertile controls. Previous studies have shown that the levels of activated macrophages in the peritoneal cavity are raised in women with endometriosis.[63–65] There appears to be an inverse relationship between severity of endometriosis and the presence of inflammatory mediators. Women with minimal-to-mild disease have higher peritoneal macrophage levels.[66,67] Cytokines secreted from endometriotic deposits or activated macrophages have been detected at higher concentrations in the peritoneal fluid of women with endometriosis and have been shown to have a detrimental effect on fertility.[68,69] There is a marked inhibitory effect of peritoneal fluid from women with mild-and-moderate endometriosis on CBF in vitro.[70] Moreover,[71] animal studies have suggested the possibility of existence of a macromolecular ovum capture inhibitor in the peritoneal fluid of women with endometriosis acting by forming a membrane over the fimbrial cilia, causing a complete loss of ovum capture activity. It is possible that a similar mechanism of deposition of filamentous material may inhibit the activity of cilia, and thus tubal transport, in women with endometriosis. Furthermore, one or more of the constituents of the proinflammatory peritoneal fluid found in women with endometriosis may affect ciliary beat directly. The factor(s) in endometriotic peritoneal fluid responsible for this reduction in CBF are unknown. Possible mediators include macrophages or their various secretion products. It is noteworthy that some recent in vitro studies have suggested that the interaction between human sperm and the tubal epithelium appears to be altered in explants of tubal epithelium from women with a diagnosis of endometriosis.[72] One might assume that a reduction in the number of free and motile sperm within the tubal lumen may reduce fertilization rates and thereby contribute to the subfertility associated with endometriosis. Although little is known about sperm–endosalpingeal interaction in humans, tubal integrins have been implicated in the process,[73] and integrin expression is known to be aberrant within the endometrium and endometriotic deposits of women with endometriosis.[74,75] Defective tubal transport of gametes and embryos may thus represent one of the mechanisms contributing to the association between endometriosis and infertility.

Smoking

There is a well-known association between ectopic pregnancy and cigarette smoking.[76] Even prenatal exposure to tobacco smoke has been suggested to increase the incidence of tubal disease, raising the possibility that tobacco smoke might have a permanent damaging effect on the developing Fallopian tubes.[77] In animal models, nicotine alters tubal motility[78] and decreases tubal blood flow.[79] Exposure of hamsters to doses of cigarette smoke within the range received by active or passive human smokers causes a small but significant increase in the secretory-to-ciliated cell ratio within the infundibulum.[80] Acute in vitro exposure of the hamster infundibulum to smoke solutions causes a rapid reduction in CBF, which is reversible upon washout of the smoke solution.[81] Oocyte cumulus pickup rate by the hamster oviduct is inhibited in a dose-dependent manner by smoke solutions, and this effect is not easily reversed by washout of the solution, demonstrating that the effect of smoking on ovum pickup is separate to the effect on CBF. The likely explanation for this is that smoke solutions disrupt the adhesion between the negatively charged tips of the cilia and the oocyte cumulus complex, probably by the binding of an as-yet-undetermined smoke component.[82] Animal data demonstrating reduced efficacy of ovum pickup and delayed transport along the tube because of decreased CBF may explain the higher rates of infertility and ectopic gestation seen in women who smoke. In a study involving gamete intrafallopian transfer (GIFT), no differences were found among active, passive, and nonsmokers in number of oocytes retrieved; however, the number of live births after GIFT was significantly lower for active smokers (10.5%) than for passive smokers (23.1%) or nonsmokers (33.3%).[83]

Microorganisms and Fallopian Tube Cilia

Exposure of the human Fallopian tube epithelium in vitro to fresh isolates of *N. gonorrhoeae* and to gonococcal endotoxin results in reduction and subsequent cessation of ciliary activity. This ciliostatic effect occurs before any ultrastructural changes are apparent on scanning electron microscopy.[84] Gonococci invade the nonciliated cells of the tubal mucosa, but destroy predominantly the ciliated cells, primarily by causing sloughing.[85] Gonococcal infection of the human Fallopian tube mucosa results in production of tumor necrosis factor (TNF)-α by the mucosa. The extent of loss of ciliated cells from the tubal epithelium correlates with the mucosal tissue concentration of TNF-α[86] and blocking gonococcal production of TNF-α limits epithelial damage.[87]

The association between chlamydia infection and tubal factor infertility is well recognized. Obstruction of the tubal passage would clearly cause infertility; however, in the absence of a significant mechanical distortion to the tubal anatomy, the exact mechanism by which chlamydia affects the tubal function is not fully understood. Salpingitis is associated with deciliation, which can be extensive.[88–90] It is possible that the function of the remaining cilia may not be affected.[91] In women with tubal infertility, serological evidence of chlamydial infection is not associated with changes in CBF. However, there is preliminary evidence that particular chlamydial serotypes, such as serotypes C and E, may be associated with zero or reduced levels of CBF, respectively, although the numbers of subjects sampled are small and these results must be interpreted with caution.[92] CBF is significantly lower in the surviving cilia of Fallopian tubes showing evidence of edema, erythema, or distal obstruction.[92,93] Therefore, it is possible that chlamydia causes deciliation and the associated chronic inflammation reduces CBF, although certain serotypes may affect CBF directly and may present a particularly poor prognosis for subsequent fertility.

FUTURE DIRECTIONS

A better understanding of the regulatory mechanisms influencing the tubal transport, gained through proteomic and genomic studies, would be of enormous importance in developing new diagnostic tools and therapeutic modalities for a variety of tube-related pathologies such as tubal infertility, ectopic pregnancy, and pelvic inflammatory disease.

REFERENCES

1. Talo A, Brundin J. Muscular activity in the rabbit oviduct: a combination of electric and mechanic recordings. *Biol Reprod.* 1971;**5**(1):67–77.
2. Daniel EE, Lucien P, Posey VA, Paton DM. A functional analysis of the myogenic control systems of the human Fallopian tube. *Am J Obstet Gynecol.* 1975a;**15;121**(8):1046–53.
3. Daniel EE, Posey VA, Paton DM. A structural analysis of the myogenic control systems of the human Fallopian tube. *Am J Obstet Gynecol.* 1975b;**15;121**(8):1054–66.
4. Brundin J. Pharmacology of the oviduct. In: Hafez ESE, Blandau RJ, editors. *The mammalian oviduct.* Chicago: University of Chicago Press; 1969. pp. 261–9.
5. Talo A. How the myosalpinx works in gamete and embryo transport. *Archivos de biologia y Medicina Experimentales.* 1991;**24**:361–75.
6. Talo A, Pulkkinen MO. Electrical activity in the human oviduct during the menstrual cycle. *Am J Obstet Gynecol.* 1982;**15;142**(2):135–47.
7. Hodgson BJ, Talo A, Pauerstein CJ. Oviductal ovum surrogate movement: interrelation with muscular activity. *Biol Reprod.* 1977;**16**(3):394–6.
8. Helm G, Owman C, Sjoberg NO, Walles B. Motor activity of the human Fallopian tube in vitro in relation to plasma concentration of oestradiol and progesterone, and the influence of noradrenaline. *J Reprod Fertil.* 1982;**64**(1):233–42.
9. Reinecke M. Neurotensin in the human Fallopian tube: immunohistochemical localization and effects of synthetic neurotensin on motor activity in vitro. *Neurosci Lett.* 1987;**73**(3):220–4.
10. Croxatto HB. Physiology of gamete and embryo transport through the Fallopian tube. *Reprod Biomed Online.* 2002;**4**(2):160–9.
11. Huang JC, Arbab F, Tumbusch KJ, Goldsby JS, Matijevic-Aleksic N, Wu KK. Human Fallopian tubes express prostacyclin (PGI) synthase and cyclo-oxygenases and synthesize abundant PGI. *J Clin Endocrinol Metab.* 2002;**87**(9):4361–8.
12. Downing SJ, Tay JI, Maguiness SD, Watson A, Leese HJ. Effect of inflammatory mediators on the physiology of the human Fallopian tube. *Hum Fertil* (Camb). 2002;**5**(2):54–60.
13. Ekerhovd E, Norstrom A. Involvement of a nitric oxide-cyclic guanosine monophosphate pathway in control of Fallopian tube contractility. *Gynecol Endocrinol.* 2004;**19**(5):239–46.
14. Bahathiq A, Stewart RL, Wells M, Pacey AA, Moore H, Ledger W. Production of activins by the human endosalpinx. *Journal of Clinical Endocrinology and Metabolism.* 2002;**87**:5283–9.
15. Halbert SA, Tam PY, Blandau RJ. Egg transport in the rabbit oviduct: the roles of cilia and muscle. *Science.* 1976;**12;191**(4231):1052–3.
16. Halbert SA, Becker DR, Szal SE. Ovum transport in the rat oviductal ampulla in the absence of muscle contractility. *Biol Reprod.* 1989;**40**(6):1131–6.
17. Afzelius BA, Camner P, Mossberg B. On the function of cilia in the female reproductive tract. *Fertil Steril.* 1978;**29**(1):72–4.
18. Pedersen H. Absence of dynein arms in endometrial cilia: cause of infertility? *Acta Obstet Gynecol Scand.* 1983;**62**(6):625–7.
19. Lurie M, Tur-Kaspa I, Weill S, Katz I, Rabinovici J, Goldenberg S. Ciliary ultrastructure of respiratory and Fallopian tube epithelium in a sterile woman with Kartagener's syndrome. A quantitative estimation. *Chest.* 1989:**95**(3):578–81.
20. Bleau G, Richer CL, Bousquet D. Absence of dynein arms in cilia of endocervical cells in a fertile woman. *Fertil Steril.* 1978;**30**(3):362–3.
21. McComb P, Langley L, Villalon M, Verdugo P. The oviductal cilia and Kartagener's syndrome. *Fertil Steril.* 1986 Sep;**46**(3):412–16.
22. Halbert SA, Patton DL, Zarutskie PW, Soules MR. Function and structure of cilia in the Fallopian tube of an infertile woman with Kartagener's syndrome. *Hum Reprod.* 1997;**12**(1):55–8.

23. Van's Gravesande KS, Omran H. Primary ciliary dyskinesia: clinical presentation, diagnosis, and genetics. *Ann Med.* 2005;**37**(6):439–49.
24. Zariwala MA, Knowles MR, Omran H. Genetic defects in ciliary structure and function. *Annu Rev Physiol.* 2007;**69**:423–50.
25. Morillas HN, Zariwala M, Knowles MR. Genetic causes of bronchiectasis: primary ciliary dyskinesia. *Respiration.* 2007;**74**(3):252–63.
26. Guichard C, Harricane MC, Lafitte JJ, Godard P, Zaegel M, Tack V, et al. Axonemal dynein intermediate-chain gene (DNAI1) mutations result in situs inversus and primary ciliary dyskinesia (Kartagener syndrome). *Am J Hum Genet.* 2001;**68**(4):1030–5.
27. Bartoloni L, Blouin JL, Pan Y, Gehrig C, Maiti AK, Scamuffa N, Rossier C, Jorissen M, Armengot M, Meeks M, Mitchison HM, Chung EM, Delozier-Blanchet CD, Craigen WJ, Antonarakis SE. Mutations in the DNAH11 (axonemal heavy chain dynein type 11) gene cause one form of situs inversus totalis and most likely primary ciliary dyskinesia. *Proc Natl Acad Sci U S A.* 2002;**6**;**99**(16):10282–6.
28. Hornef N, Olbrich H, Horvath J, Zariwala MA, Fliegauf M, Loges NT, et al. DNAH5 mutations are a common cause of primary ciliary dyskinesia with outer dynein arm defects. *Am J Respir Crit Care Med.* 2006;**15**;**174**(2):120–6.
29. Verdugo P. Ca2+-dependent hormonal stimulation of ciliary activity. *Nature.* 1980; **283**:764–5.
30. Villalon M, Cardina-Danovaro M. ATP increases the frequency of ciliary beat of human oviductal ciliated cells. *Prog Clin Biol Res.* 1994;**80**:59–65.
31. Verdugo P, Johnson NT, Tam PY. Beta-adrenergic stimulation of respiratory ciliary activity. *J Appl Physiol.* 1980b;**48**:868–71.
32. Saridogan E, Djahanbakhch O, Puddefoot JR, Demetroulis C, Collingwood K, Mehta JG, et al. Angiotensin II receptors and angiotensin II stimulation of ciliary activity in human Fallopian tube. *J Clin Endocrinol Metab.* 1996;**81**(7):2719–25.
33. Jansen RP. Endocrine response in the Fallopian tube. *Endocr Rev.* 1984;**5**(4):525–51.
34. Mahmood T, Saridogan E, Smutna S, Habib AM, Djahanbakhch O. The effect of ovarian steroids on epithelial ciliary beat frequency in the human Fallopian tube. *Hum Reprod.* 1998;**13**(11):2991–4.
35. Paltieli Y, Eibschitz I, Ziskind G, Ohel G, Silbermann M, Weichselbaum A. High progesterone levels and ciliary dysfunction: a possible cause of ectopic pregnancy. *J Assist Reprod Genet.* 2000;**17**:103–6.
36. Bendz A, Hansson HA, Svendsen P, Wiqvist N. On the extensive contact between veins and arteries in the human ovarian pedicle. *Acta Physiol Scand.* 1982;**115**:179–82.
37. Lyons RA, Djahanbakhch O, Mahmood T, Saridogan E, Sattar S, Sheaff MT, et al. Fallopian tube ciliary beat frequency in relation to the stage of menstrual cycle and anatomical site. *Hum Reprod.* 2002a;**17**:584–8.
38. Lyons RA, Saridogan E, Djahanbakhch O. The reproductive significance of human Fallopian tube cilia. *Hum Reprod Update.* 2006b;**12**(4):363–72.
39. Verdugo P, Rumery RE, Tam PY. Hormonal control of oviductal ciliary activity: effect of prostaglandins. *Fertil Steril.* 1980a;**33**:193–6.
40. Lyons RA, Saridogan E, Djahanbakhch O. The effect of ovarian follicular fluid and peritoneal fluid on Fallopian tube ciliary beat frequency. *Hum Reprod.* 2006a; **21**(1):52–6.
41. Edwards RG, Steptoe PC, Abraham GE, Walters E, Purdy JM, Fotherby K. Steroid assays and preovulatory follicular development in human ovaries primed with gonadotrophins. *Lancet.* 1972;**2**:611–15.
42. McNatty KP, Smith DM, Makris A, Osathanondh R, Ryan KJ. The microenvironment of the human antral follicle: interrelationships among the steroid levels in antral fluid, the population of granulosa cells, and the status of the oocyte in vivo and in vitro. *J Clin Endocrinol Metab.* 1979;**49**:851–60.
43. Seibel MM, Swartz SL, Smith D, Levesque L, Taymor ML. In vivo prostaglandin concentrations in human preovulatory follicles. *Fertil Steril.* 1984;**42**:482–5.

44. Doyle JB. Tubo-ovarian mechanism; observation at laparotomy. *Obstet Gynecol.* 1956; **8**:686–90.
45. Harper MJK. Sperm and egg transport. In: Austin CR, Short RV, editors. *Germ cells and fertilization*, 2nd ed. Cambridge, UK: Cambridge University Press; 1982. pp. 102–27.
46. Lindblom B, Norström A. The smooth muscle architecture of the human Fallopian tube. In: Siegler AM, editor. *The Fallopian tube. basic studies and clinical contributions.* Mount Kisco: Futura Publishing Co., Inc.; 1986. pp. 13–20.
47. Okamura H, Morikawa H, Oshima M, Man-i M, Nishimura T. A morphologic study of mesotubarium ovarica in the human. *Obstet Gynecol.* 1977;**49**:197–201.
48. Edwards RG, Steptoe PC. Induction of follicular growth, ovulation, and luteinization in the human ovary. *J Reprod Fertil.* 1975;**22**(Suppl):121–63.
49. Sterin-Speziale N, Gimeno MF, Zapata C, Bagnati PE, Gimeno AL. The effect of neurotransmitters, bradykinin, prostaglandins, and follicular fluid on spontaneous contractile characteristics of human fimbria and tubo-ovarian ligaments isolated during different stages of the sexual cycle. *Int J Fertil.* 1978;**23**:1–11.
50. Morikawa H, Okamura H, Takenaka A, Morimoto K, Nishimura T. Physiological study of the human mesotubarium ovarica. *Obstet Gynecol.* 1980;**55**:493–6.
51. Gordts S, Campo R, Romauts L, Brosen I. Endoscopic visualization of the process of fimbrial ovum retrieval in the human. *Hum Reprod.* 1998;**13**:1425–8.
52. White MM, Zamudio S, Stevens T et al. Estrogen, progesterone, and vascular reactivity: potential cellular mechanisms. *Endocr Rev.* 1995;**16**:739–51.
53. Magness RR, Rosenfeld CR, Carr BR. Protein kinase C in uterine and systemic arteries during ovarian cycle and pregnancy. *Am J Physiol Endocrinol Metabol.* 1991;**260**:23–30.
54. Croxatto HB, Ortiz ME, Diaz S, Hess R, Balmaceda J, Croxatto HD. Studies on the duration of egg transport by the human oviduct. II. Ovum location at various intervals following luteinizing hormone peak. *Am J Obstet Gynecol.* 1978;**132**:629–34.
55. Croxatto HB, Ortiz ME. Egg transport in the Fallopian tube. *Gynecol Invest.* 1975;**6**:215–25.
56. Jansen RP. Cyclic changes in the human Fallopian tube isthmus and their functional importance. *Am J Obstet Gynecol.* 1980;**1**;**136**(3):292–308.
57. Anand S, Guha SK. Dynamics of the ampullary-isthmic junction in rabbit oviduct. *Gynecol Obstet Invest.* 1982;**14**:39–46.
58. Jansen RP. Fallopian tube isthmic mucus and ovum transport. *Science.* 1978;**201**:349–51.
59. Croxatto HB, Ortiz ME. Oocyte pickup and oviductal transport. In: Capitanio GL, Asch RH, De Cecco L, Croce S, editors. *GIFT: From basics to clinic.* New York: Raven Press; 1989. pp. 137–47.
60. Kleiner GJ, Roberts TW. Current factors in the causation of tubal pregnancy: a prospective clinicopathologic study. *Am J Obstet Gynecol.* 1967;**1**;**99**(1):21–8.
61. Vasquez G, Winston, RML, Brosens, IA. Tubal mucosa and ectopic pregnancy. *Br J Obstet Gynaecol.* 1983;**99**:468–74.
62. Diaz J, Vasquesz J, Diaz S, et al. Transport of ovum surrogates by the human oviduct. In: Harper MJK, Pauerstein CJ, Adams CE, et al., editors. *Ovum transport and fertility regulation.* Copenhagen: Scriptor; 1976. pp. 404–15.
63. Halme J, Becker S, Hammond MG, Raj MH, Raj S. Increased activation of pelvic macrophages in infertile women with mild endometriosis. *Am J Obstet Gynecol.* 1983;**145**:333–7.
64. Halme J, Becker S, Haskill S. Altered maturation and function of peritoneal macrophages: possible role in pathogenesis of endometriosis. *Am J Obstet Gynecol.* 1987;**156**:783–9.
65. Zeller JM, Henig I, Radwanska E, Dmowski WP. Enhancement of human monocyte and peritoneal macrophage chemiluminescence activities in women with endometriosis. *Am J Reprod Immunol Microbiol.* 1987;**13**:78–82.

66. Olive DL, Weinberg JB, Haney AF. Peritoneal macrophages and infertility: the association between cell number and pelvic pathology. *Fertil Steril.* 1985;**44**:772–7.
67. Haney AF, Jenkins S, Weinberg JB. The stimulus responsible for the peritoneal fluid inflammation observed in infertile women with endometriosis. *Fertil Steril.* 1991;**56**:408–13.
68. Fakih H, Baggett B, Holtz G, Tsang K. Interleukin-1: a possible role in the infertility associated with endometriosis. *Fertil Steril.* 1987;**47**:213–17.
69. Sueldo CE, Kelly E, Montoro L, Subias E, Baccaro M, Swanson JA, et al. Effect of interleukin–1 on gamete interaction and mouse embryo development. *J Reprod Med.* 1990;**35**:868–72.
70. Lyons RA, Djahanbakhch O, Saridogan E, Naftalin AA, Mahmood T, Weekes A, et al. Peritoneal fluid, endometriosis, and ciliary beat frequency in the human Fallopian tube. *Lancet.* 2002b;**360**(9341):1221–2.
71. Suginami H, Yano K. An ovum capture inhibitor (OCI) in endometriosis peritoneal fluid: an OCI-related membrane responsible for fimbrial failure of ovum capture. *Fertil Steril.* 1988;**50**:648–53.
72. Reeve L, Lashen H, Pacey AA. Endometriosis affects spermendosalpingeal interactions. *Hum Reprod.* 2005;**20**:448–51.
73. Reeve L, Ledger WL, Pacey AA. Does the Arg-Gly-Asp (RGD) adhesion sequence play a role in mediating sperm interaction with the human endosalpinx? *Hum Reprod.* 2003;**18**:1461–8.
74. Lessey BA, Castelbaum AJ, Sawin SW, Buck CA, Schinnar R, Bilker W, et al. Aberrant integrin expression in the endometrium of women with endometriosis. *J Clin Endocrinol Metab.* 1994;**79**:643–9.
75. Puy LA, Pang C, Librach CL. Immunohistochemical analysis of alphavbeta5 and alphavbeta6 integrins in the endometrium and endometriosis. *Int J Gynecol Pathol.* 2002;**21**:167–77.
76. Bouyer J, Coste J, Shojaei T, Pouly JL, Fernandez H, Gerbaud L, Job-Spira N. Risk factors for ectopic pregnancy: a comprehensive analysis based on a large case-control, population-based study in France. *Am J Epidemiol.* 2003;**157**:185–94.
77. Matthews SJ, Shires S, Picton HM, Rutherford AJ, Balen AH, Sharma V, et al. Pre- and post-natal tobacco exposure and tubal disease. *Hum Reprod.* 17, Abstract Book 2002;**1**:80.
78. Neri A, Marcus SL. Effect of nicotine on the motility of the oviducts in the rhesus monkey: a preliminary report. *J Reprod Fertil.* 1972;**31**:91–7.
79. Mitchell JA, Hammer RE. Effects of nicotine on oviductal blood flow and embryo development in the rat. *J Reprod Fertil.* 1985;**74**:71–6.
80. Magers T, Talbot P, DiCarlantonio G, Knoll M, Demers D, Tsai I, et al. Cigarette smoke inhalation affects the reproductive system of female hamsters. *Reprod Toxicol.* 1995;**9**(6):513–25.
81. Knoll M, Shaoulian R, Magers T, Talbot P. Ciliary beat frequency of hamster oviducts is decreased in vitro by exposure to solutions of mainstream and sidestream cigarette smoke. *Biol Reprod.* 1995;**53**:29–37.
82. Knoll M, Talbot P. Cigarette smoke inhibits oocyte cumulus complex pick-up by the oviduct in vitro independent of ciliary beat frequency. *Reprod Toxicol Jan–Feb.* 1998;**12**(1):57–68.
83. Chung PH, Yeko TR, Mayer JC, Clark B, Welden SW, Maroulis GB. Gamete intrafallopian transfer: does smoking play a role? *J Reprod Med.* 1997;**42**:65–70.
84. Mardh PA, Baldetorp B, Hakansson CH, Fritz H, Westrom L. Studies of ciliated epithelia of the human genital tract. 3: mucociliary wave activity in organ cultures of human Fallopian tubes challenged with Neisseria gonorrhoeae and gonococcal endotoxin. *Br J Vener Dis.* 1979;**55**:256–64.

85. McGee ZA, Johnson AP, Taylor-Robinson D. Pathogenic mechanisms of Neisseria gonorrhoeae: observations on damage to human Fallopian tubes in organ culture by gonococci of colony type 1 or type 4. *J Infect Dis.* 1981;**143**:413–22.
86. McGee ZA, Jensen RL, Clemens CM, Taylor-Robinson D, Johnson AP, Gregg CR. Gonococcal infection of human Fallopian tube mucosa in organ culture: relationship of mucosal tissue TNF-alpha concentration to sloughing of ciliated cells. *Sex Transm Dis.* 1999;**26**:160–5.
87. McGee ZA, Clemens CM, Jensen RL, Klein JJ, Barley LR, Gorby GL. Local induction of tumor necrosis factor as a molecular mechanism of mucosal damage by gonococci. *Microb Pathog.* 1992;**12**:333–41.
88. Patton DL, Halbert SA, Kuo CC, Wang SP, Holmes KK. Host response to primary Chlamydia trachomatis infection of the Fallopian tube in pig-tailed monkeys. *Fertil Steril.* 1983;**40**:829–40.
89. Patton DL, Kuo CC, Wang SP, Halbert SA. Distal tubal obstruction induced by repeated Chlamydia trachomatis salpingeal infections in pigtailed macaques. *J Infect Dis.* 1987;**155**:1292–9.
90. Westrom L, Wolner-Hanssen P. Pathogenesis of pelvic inflammatory disease. *Genitourin Med.* 1993;**69**:9–17.
91. Cooper MD, Rapp J, Jeffery-Wiseman C, Barnes RC, Stephens DS. Chlamydia trachomatis infection of human Fallopian tube organ cultures. *J Gen Microbiol.* 1990;**136**:1109–15.
92. Leng Z, Moore DE, Mueller BA, Critchlow CW, Patton DL, Halbert SA, Wang SP. Characterization of ciliary activity in distal Fallopian tube biopsies of women with obstructive tubal infertility. *Hum Reprod.* 1998;**13**:3121–7.
93. Patton DL, Moore DE, Spadoni LR, Soules MR, Halbert SA, Wang SP. A comparison of the Fallopian tube's response to overt and silent salpingitis. *Obstet Gynecol.* 1989;**73**:622–30.

IV

INFECTIONS AND INFLAMMATORY CAUSES OF TUBAL INFERTILITY

Adrian R. Eley and Ying C. Cheong

CHLAMYDIA TRACHOMATIS – AN INTRODUCTION

Chlamydia trachomatis is an obligate, intracellular Gram-negative bacterium that is characterized by a unique developmental cycle. This consists of an infectious form, the elementary body (EB), which after attachment to the host and internalization, differentiates to become the replicative form, the reticulate body (RB). After multiplication, the RBs turn back into EBs and these are then released to begin the cycle again (Fig. 4.1).

There is a certain amount of controversy as to how *C. trachomatis* attaches to the host and what the host receptor or receptors are.[1,2] However, electron microscopic studies have clearly shown that EBs interact directly with the host epithelium, with possible encirclement by microvilli, before internalization and the induction of the inflammatory process (Fig. 4.2).

Chlamydial isolates are usually differentiated into serovars based on antigenic variation of the major outer membrane protein (MOMP). Serovars D to K and L1 to L3 are sexually transmitted pathogens, which typically cause urethritis and cervicitis or lymphogranuloma venereum (LGV), respectively.

Chlamydia trachomatis is now widely believed to be the cause of the most prevalent bacterial sexually transmitted infections worldwide and is particularly common among persons under age 25, living in industrialized nations. The organism is widely seen in the United States and the rest of the Western world including the United Kingdom, where the number of infections has risen rapidly in the last few years (Fig. 4.3). In developed countries the prevalence of chlamydial infection is reported to be about 3 percent in the general population.[3] In developing countries, however, the prevalence is considerably higher among sexually active women. A serological study in the West Indies showed that 32 percent of pregnant women had a titer of $\geq$512 in the whole inclusion immunofluorescence (WHIF) test for *C. trachomatis*.[4]

One of the major difficulties in clinical practice working with patients with suspected chlamydial disease has been the problem of laboratory diagnosis. More recently, however, molecular diagnostics such as the use of nucleic acid amplification tests (NAATs) have been introduced as routine procedures, which have improved both sensitivity and specificity. Such tests have been used in research studies into tubal damage caused by *C. trachomatis* and have been instrumental in helping us understand the magnitude of the problem.[5] However, more routine testing in fertility assessment involves detection of *C. trachomatis* antibodies because there is a possible link between serological evidence of previous

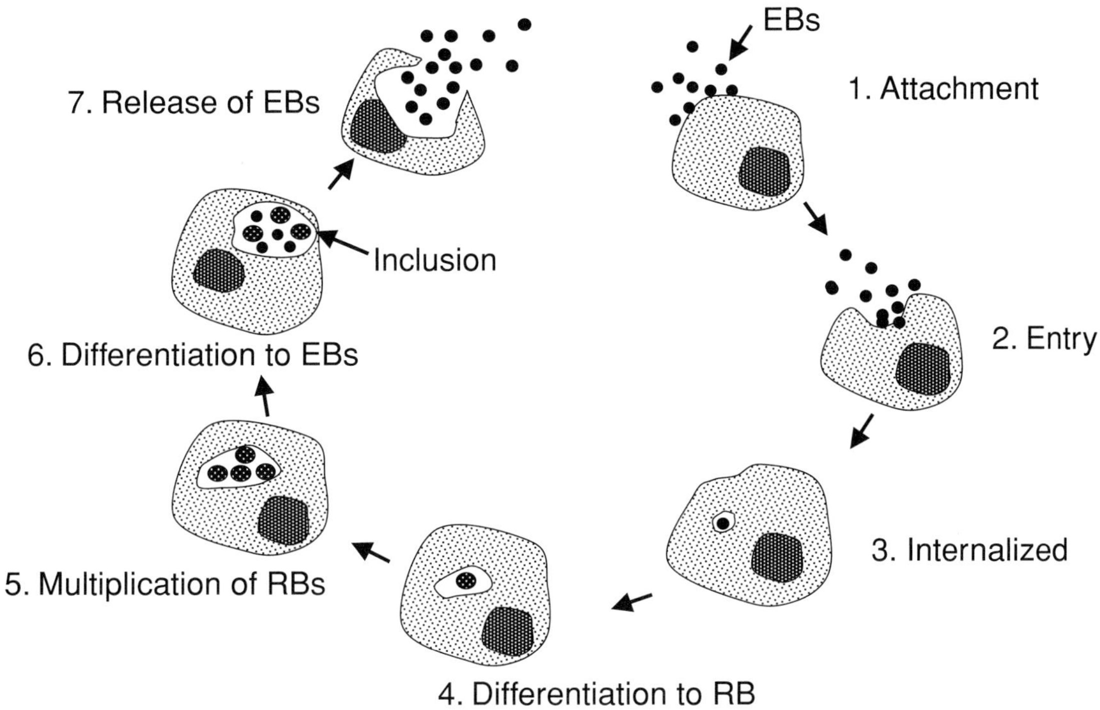

Fig. 4.1: Developmental cycle of *Chlamydia trachomatis*.

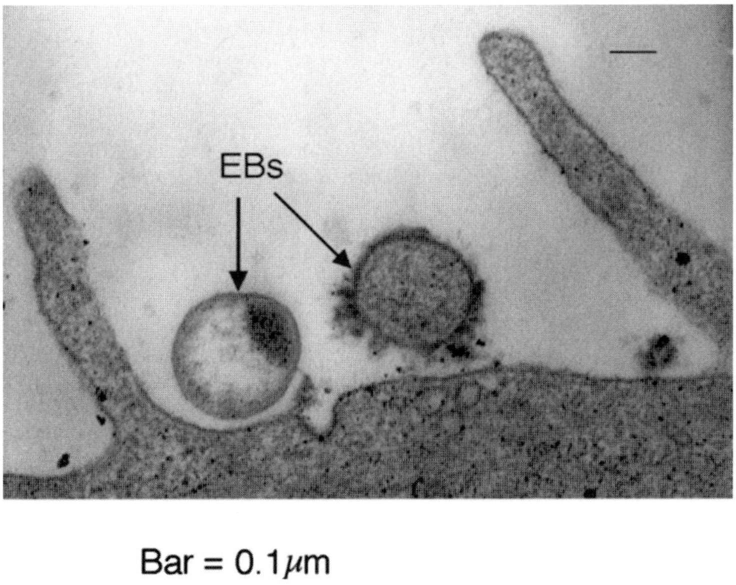

Fig. 4.2: Electron microscopy showing elementary bodies (EBs) in the first stages of adherence to the host epithelium.

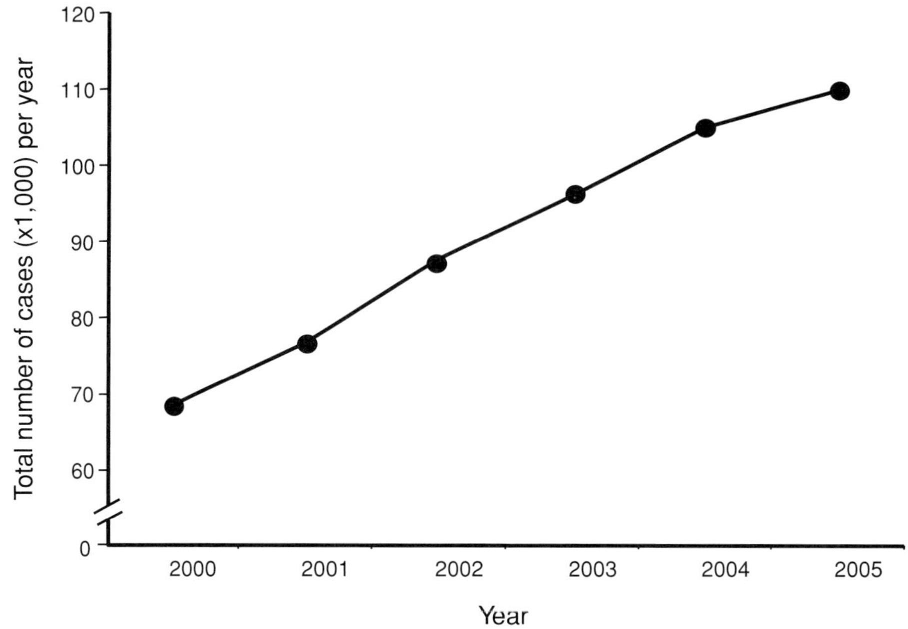

Fig 4.3: Uncomplicated genital chlamydial infections in UK, 2000–2005.

C. trachomatis infections and tubal factor infertility (TFI).[6] An example is the use of an **e**nzyme **l**inked **i**mmuno**s**orbent **a**ssay (ELISA) with antigen-coated wells in a microtiter plate, which produces a color change of a substrate in the presence of the patient's antibody. Despite the disadvantages of ELISA testing that include reduced specificity and sensitivity, many samples can be performed on a single microtiter plate (Fig. 4.4).

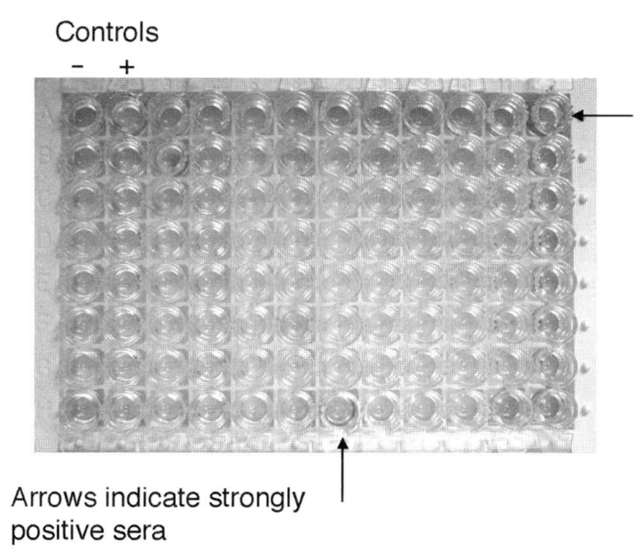

Fig. 4.4: ELISA showing detection of chlamydial antibodies on a microtitre plate. (See Color Plate 3.)

With an increasing prevalence of *C. trachomatis* in the UK and because routine antibiotic treatment is both cheap and generally effective in the management of lower genital tract infections, a national chlamydia screening program has been introduced. The aim of the program, which is targeted to the younger population, is to detect the organism and provide treatment to reduce the future burden of tubal damage. Previous screening programs in Scandinavia and the United States have shown that sequelae of chronic chlamydial infections can be significantly reduced. If the UK screening program is effective, then in the future, the increasing risk of tubal damage should be curtailed.[7,8]

THE ROLE OF *C. TRACHOMATIS* IN THE FEMALE GENITAL TRACT

Acute *C. trachomatis* infection is a frequent cause of mucopurulent but often asymptomatic cervicitis in women. If the organism ascends to the upper genital tract in women, it can result in severe complications such as pelvic inflammatory disease (PID), ectopic pregnancy, pelvic adhesions, and TFI. The clinical spectrum of *C. trachomatis* PID is broad and includes endometritis, salpingitis, tubo-ovarian abscess, pelvic peritonitis, periappendicitis, and perihepatitis.

It is widely known that repeated and/or persistent chlamydial infections (which may last for years) are particularly associated with pathology. For example, in young women, recurrent genital tract infections were associated with an increased risk of PID.[9] Moreover, in another study, each episode of PID roughly doubled the risk of permanent tubal damage.[10] Repeated genital tract infections were necessary to produce the pelvic adhesions, tubal scarring, and occlusion characteristic of severe PID.[11] However, the situation is not clear-cut because not all women infected with *C. trachomatis* go on to develop sequelae such as tubal pathology.[12]

What is known is that *C. trachomatis* infection is the most important cause of tubal pathology, with 296.5 cases per 100,000 population reported in the United States in 2002.[13] Using different techniques, between 50 and 70 percent of TFI cases may be caused by *C. trachomatis.*[5,14] In the upper genital tract following chlamydial infection, the worst-case scenario is that inflammation follows, which is exacerbated by reinfection and may ultimately lead to tissue damage and scarring. This has been reproduced in an animal model using guinea pigs and the *Chlamydophila psittaci* guinea-pig inclusion conjunctivitis (GPIC) agent. Early on there is an acute inflammatory response followed by chronic inflammation, which is enhanced by repeated infections resulting in increased oviduct damage.[15] Long-term fibrosis occurred in approximately 20 percent of the animals tested.

There is no doubt that the precise pathogenesis of tubal damage caused by *C. trachomatis* infection remains to be elucidated. Nevertheless, immunopathology of tubal chlamydial infections may in part depend on the virulence of the organism but perhaps more importantly on differences in host factors such as genetic polymorphisms as discussed next.

The HLA systems control immune responses by presenting antigenic epitopes to immune T cells. HLA molecules regulate the range of immune responses to different antigens and mediate susceptibility or resistance to infecting microorganisms. *C. trachomatis*–associated PID has been linked with the HLA-A31 gene,[16] whereas *C. trachomatis*-associated TFI has been linked with HLA-DQA*0101 and DQB*0501 alleles.[17] A more recent study of women with chlamydial TFI has shown an association with the IL-10–1082AA and the HLA-DQA1*0102 and DQB1*0602 alleles that was related to a lymphocyte proliferative response to CHSP60 antigen.[18] This suggests that the CHSP60–associated immune response (which will be discussed later) may be linked with the host's genetic factors. Another recent development has focused on CCR5, a chemokine receptor involved in T-cell activation and function. In women with positive antichlamydial IgG responses, a low incidence of CCR5delta32 deletion correlated with tubal pathology while a high incidence was seen in women without tubal pathology.[19] This suggests that inflammation associated with CCR5 function may predispose women to development of complications of chlamydial infection, such as TFI. In contrast, the Asp299 Glu single nucleotide polymorphism of human TLR4, which is the most commonly described, was shown to have played no part in susceptibility to *C. trachomatis*–associated tubal infertility.[20] However, it was pointed out that the serological tests for *C. trachomatis* used in the study were suboptimal and could have been improved, thereby raising doubts as to the validity of the work.[21] Another possibility for some chlamydial infections being more damaging than others is that there are differences in the pathogen itself. Evidence from a long-term persistence study showed that the majority of women with recurrent infection were infected with more unusual serovars (J, Ia, K, or H instead of D, E, or F, which are the most common).[22] This suggests that there may be a tendency for certain serovars to be more pathogenic. However, when genetic studies on individual virulence factors have been examined in more detail, apart from polymorphisms in the *C. trachomatis* cytotoxin locus being associated with disease, the findings have been disappointing.[23,24]

When *C. trachomatis* infects host epithelial cells in the upper genital tract, this can evoke peritonitis whereby proinflammatory cytokines are being produced by both the tubal epithelial cells and the peritoneum, which may result in peritubal, periovarian pelvic adhesions (see Fig. 4.7). Chlamydial infection can also generate a cytokine response by interaction with cells of the immune system. Recent evidence from a cell coculture model suggests that interleukins-6 and 8 (IL-6, IL-8) in particular may be involved in the immunopathogenesis of chronic chlamydial infections.[25] Other cytokines such as granulocyte-macrophage colony-stimulating factor (GM-CSF), interleukins 1-α, 10, and 12 (IL-1α, IL-10, IL-12) have also been detected following chlamydial infection. In in vitro studies, another proinflammatory cytokine, gamma interferon (IFN-γ), has been shown to be important in pathogenesis. It is also known as a precursor to fibrosis, scarring, and sequelae, and as a potent inducer of the incomplete chlamydial developmental cycle, which can lead to persistence and the upregulation of chlamydial heat shock protein.[26]

Table 4.1 Different Serological Markers Used to Predict Tubal Damage in Infertile Women

Markers	*References*
C. trachomatis IgG antibodies	Mouton et al.[44]
C. trachomatis IgA antibodies	Mouton et al.[44]
C. trachomatis HSP60 IgG antibodies	Dadamessi et al.[28]
C. trachomatis HSP10 IgG antibodies	Dadamessi et al.[28]
Chlamydial lipopolysaccharide IgG antibodies	Persson et al.[45]
C-reactive protein (<10 mg/l)*	den Hartog et al.[27]
Lymphocyte proliferation assay†	Tiitinen et al.[14]

* Preferably in combination with *C. trachomatis* IgG antibodies.
† Preferably in combination with *C. trachomatis* HSP60 IgG antibodies.

Heat Shock Proteins

Heat shock proteins are a family of proteins widely distributed in almost all organisms that are expressed as a result of exposure of an organism to stress. Such stresses could include inflamed or damaged tissue caused by *C. trachomatis*. Perhaps the most common chlamydial heat shock protein produced is CHSP60, which relates to the protein's molecular weight (60 kDa).

The theory is that immune responses to microbial heat shock proteins, especially HSP60, might initiate an immune response against the related human heat shock protein through antigenic mimicry. A significant development from this finding has been the association between antibodies to CHSP60 and the chronic sequelae of chlamydial infection.[14,27,28]

Screening

Despite the fact that routine serological screening for previous *C. trachomatis* infection lacks sensitivity and accuracy, ideally a simple, reliable, and cost-effective test for *C. trachomatis*-related tubal damage among infertile women would be useful and could influence further patient management. Interestingly, a number of serological markers have been used to determine different antibody responses (Table 4.1), and their use in predicting tubal damage can be improved by combining tests.[14,27,28] Nevertheless, opinions differ widely on the usefulness of serological testing. In one study, serology failed to predict tubal damage in subfertile women while another study showed that the serum chlamydial antibody level is a useful tool for predicting the severity of tubal disease.[29,30]

The most recent evidence shows that predictions about tubal damage can be improved by combining tests for both humoral and cell-mediated immune (CMI) responses to chlamydial antigens. Although there are no current commercial tests for these CMI responses, there is some evidence that immunogenesis of tubal damage also involves cell-mediated mechanisms[31,32] giving some credence to the reasoning behind combining tests for humoral and CMI responses.

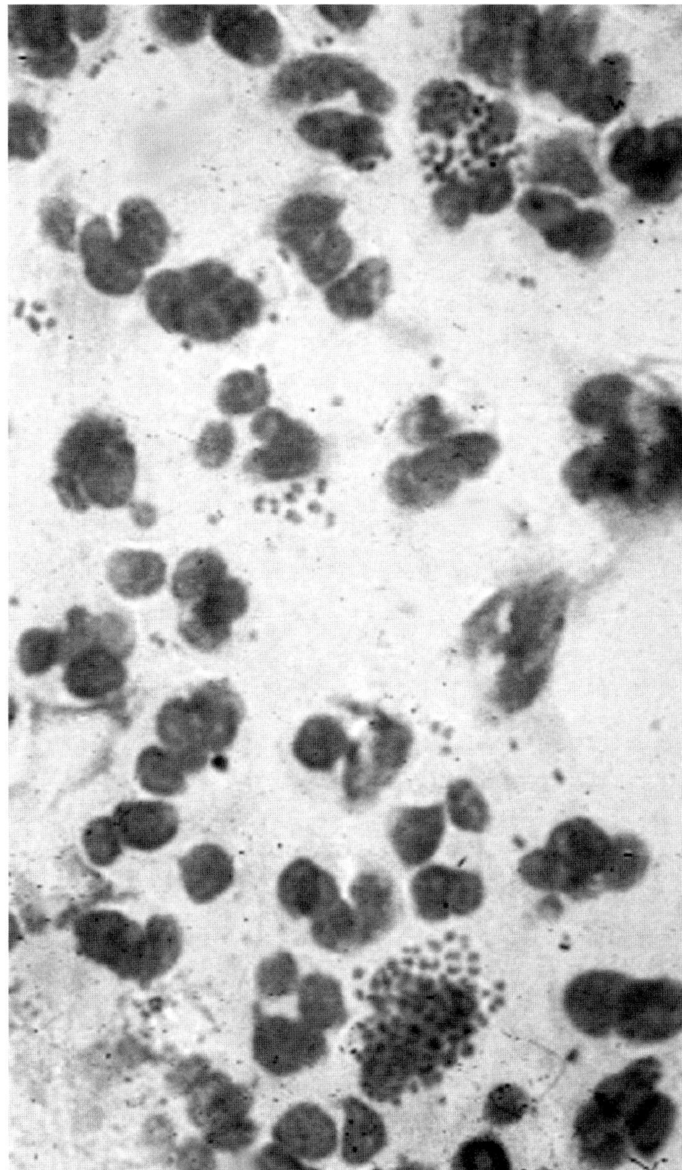

Fig. 4.5: Gram stain of *Neisseria gonorrhoeae*. (See Color Plate 4.)

Gonorrhea and Tubal Disease

Neisseria gonorrhoeae is the etiological agent of gonorrhea and is commonly known as the gonococcus. It is a Gram-negative diplococcus (Fig. 4.5), which causes the sexually transmitted disease gonorrhea. It has also been known as "the clap" for a long time and like many words, it has changed just enough over the years to obscure its origins. However, the slang may originate from the French word *clapoir*, which refers to a sexual sore, and dates back as far as 1587.

In comparison to chlamydial infection, gonorrhea is far less prevalent. The prevalence of *N. gonorrhoeae* peaked after World War II but unlike chlamydial infections, its prevalence in industrialized countries has declined steadily in recent years.[33] A wide range of prevalence rates for gonorrhea among STD clinic patients has been documented: 1 to 5 percent in Western European countries and Australia and 15 percent in the United States.[34] A UK prospective longitudinal cohort study involving 104 women with laparoscopically diagnosed salpingitis (inflammation of one or both of the Fallopian tubes) identified *C. trachomatis* in 39 percent of women and *N. gonorrhoeae* in 14 percent of women. In the study group, nearly 8 percent of women were coinfected with chlamydia and *N gonorrhoeae.*[35]

The primary sites of infection are the mucous membranes of the urethra, endocervix, rectum, pharynx, and conjunctiva. Transmission is by direct inoculation of secretions from one mucous membrane to another. Although the majority of infected men have symptoms such as urethral discharge (80%) and dysuria (50%), up to 50 percent of women infected will remain asymptomatic. When untreated, gonorrhea may progress locally to cause PID in females, epididymitis, and orchitis in males, and sterility in both sexes. PID, especially if recurrent, often causes decreased fertility, can lead to tubo-ovarian abscess, and, rarely, tubal perforation with peritonitis and death. Females with recurrent PID have high rates of ectopic pregnancy and infertility: approximately 8 percent after one episode, 20 percent after two episodes, and 40 percent after three or more episodes. PID with either *N. gonorrhoeae* or *C. trachomatis* can lead to perihepatitis and the classic Fitz-Hugh-Curtis syndrome where violin string-like adhesions can be visualized during laparoscopy between the anterior abdominal wall and the anterior surface of the liver.

Studies reveal that the gonococcus can enter human cells, but only recently has it been shown that the organism is intracellular during human infection. A repertoire of virulence factors has been identified that allow this bacterium to successfully adapt to variable microenvironments within its sole host, the human. This human adaptability and the repeated phase and antigenic change displayed by the gonococcus have hampered vaccine development. It has been demonstrated that gonococci attach specifically to nonciliated cells and that attachment is mediated by both pili and Opa (opacity-related) protein.[36] Following the attachment of the bacteria, ciliated cells are damaged, thus leading to sloughing of cells from the epithelium and a loss of ciliary activity. It is thought that the bacterial components that mediate this damage are lipo-oligosaccharide and fragments of peptidoglycan. However, the nature of the inflammatory mediators induced following gonococcal interactions is poorly understood. Challenging explants of human Fallopian tubes with gonococci has been shown to induce mRNA expression and protein secretion for the proinflammatory cytokines IL-1 and TNF-α.[37] Cell surface receptors for TNF-α are widely distributed among different tissues, and many cell types express both TNF-R1 and TNF-RII. The cytoplasm of TNF-RI has a "death domain," which has been reported to trigger an apoptotic pathway,[38] and Maisey et al.[37] hypothesized that it is possible that this mechanism is induced in the mucosal epithelium of a Fallopian tube infected with gonococci. Therefore, cytotoxicity resulting from the effects of TNF-α, acting in concert with TNF receptors on the mucosal epithelium, may be host-protective during the initial infection in limiting penetration of the organism to submucosal tissue. Similarly, studies using distinct epithelial cell lines from normal human endocervix, ectocervix, and vagina demonstrated the ability of gonococci to stimulate a distinct proinflammatory response involving the upregulation of IL-8, IL-6, and intercellular adhesion molecule 1 (CD54).[39] The release of proinflammatory cytokines and the resultant inflammatory changes because of infection can lead to intratubal as well as peritubal/pelvic adhesion formation, with consequent mechanical and functional tubal blockage. In a subset of women from the PEACH (PID Evaluation and Clinical Health) study, Ness et al.[39] have found that chlamydial and gonococcal cervicitis, endometritis, and tubal infertility were more common among women carrying the HLA class II DQA*301 allele (see previous section on *C. trachomatis*). Conversely, pregnancy was more common among women carrying DQA*0501 and DQB*0402 alleles.[39]

As for laboratory diagnosis, culture is the most common test, although NAATs as in testing for *C. trachomatis* have become popular. A culture or nonculture detection test for *N. gonorrhoeae* is usually performed on endocervical, urethral, pharyngeal, or rectal swabs. Because organisms are intracellular, one needs to obtain a more clinically invasive specimen in a manner that will contain mucosal cells and not merely discharge (similar to a Papanicolaou smear). Importantly, nonculture tests are less accurate in the presence of blood or during menses. Culture can be performed on a medium such as Thayer-Martin agar, which must be incubated in an atmosphere with increased carbon dioxide. Culture offers a readily available, sensitive (>95%), and cheap diagnostic test that also has the advantage of allowing antimicrobial sensitivity testing. It is currently the choice of testing in the UK when more than simply detection is required.

Current recommended treatment includes ciprofloxacin, ofloxacin, or spectinomycin. As always, antimicrobial therapy should take into account local patterns of antimicrobial susceptibility of the gonococcus. There is currently no strong evidence available to suggest that universal or targeted screening strategies for this infection are cost-effective as the prevalence of gonococcal disease is typically less than chlamydial infection. However, recent evidence only addresses key questions about risk factors and new tests, but the studies were limited by descriptive, cross-sectional designs focusing on highly prevalent communities and settings, such as specific clinics, and therefore cannot be generalized to primary care.

Tuberculosis and Tubal Disease

Tuberculosis (TB) is a chronic bacterial infection caused by *Mycobacterium tuberculosis*, and discovered by Koch in 1882. Cell-mediated hypersensitivity is a characteristic of TB. Genital tuberculosis is nearly always secondary to a primary focus elsewhere in the body, but the spread takes place at an early stage of the disease. Autopsy studies reveal that 4 to 12 percent of women who have died of pulmonary tuberculosis also have evidence of genital tract involvement.[40] Fallopian tube involvement is evident in most cases. The tubes may appear normal on external appearance or may show a hydrosalpinx, a pyosalpinx, or even calcification. Adhesions around the Fallopian tubes and ovaries are seen in most cases. Ovarian involvement may lead to formation of tubo-ovarian masses. Although tuberculosis is a common cause of infertility in developing countries and in Asia in particular, its rarity as a cause of infertility in the UK has led to the diagnosis often being missed. Infertility is often one of the symptoms and sometimes the only reason to investigate for the presence of the condition. Pelvic tuberculosis usually presents with one or more of the following signs and symptoms:

- Pelvic pain: dysmenorrhea, dyspareunia, chronic lower abdominal pain or discomfort, and chronic backache
- Abdominal distention: this is usually due to ascites (collection of free fluid in the abdominal-pelvic cavity)
- Infertility: most commonly due to tuberculous salpingitis (tubal disease), ovulation dysfunction that often presents with absent, excessive, or noncyclical menstruation, largely attributable to ovarian involvement and uterine (endometrial) tuberculosis.

Local tuberculous lesions may appear in the cervix and vagina. The diagnosis is made on the basis of clinical suspicion where there is evidence of concomitant pulmonary tuberculosis, the detection of calcifications on pelvic X-rays, or a typical tubal pattern on hysterosalpingogram (HSG). Occasionally the findings during surgery and the subsequent pathological and microbiological examination of biopsy material obtained during these procedures help with the diagnosis. Management is primarily directed toward the eradication of the infection by means of specific chemotherapeutics such as para-aminosalicylic acid (PAS), isoniazid (INH), rifampicin, and streptomycin derivatives. Pelvic surgery (other than to remove distended or infected lesions and damaged Fallopian tubes) has little therapeutic benefit. Provided that the tuberculous process has not destroyed the uterine lining, in vitro fertilization (IVF) following successful antibacterial treatment is the only rational method of treating infertility associated with pelvic tuberculosis.

There are many new approaches for discovering more selective anti-TB agents: the mapping of the *M. tuberculosis* genome; the delineation of many of the pathways in mycobacterial cell wall biosynthesis (e.g., glycosylation pathways, fatty acid biosynthesis, and diaminopimelic acid biosynthesis); the discovery of genes involved in latency and virulence; and the application of DNA microarray technology to *M. tuberculosis*. Furthermore, the application of combinatorial chemistry and high-throughput screening to anti-TB drug discovery promises to greatly accelerate the drug discovery process.

Crohn's Disease

Crohn's disease is a chronic inflammatory disorder of unknown etiology that may involve any portion of the gastrointestinal tract. Transmural inflammation penetrating directly into adjacent organs is common in Crohn's disease, and internal fistulas have been reported in as many as one-third of patients. In rare instances, Crohn's disease is a cause of granulomatous lesions involving the Fallopian tubes or the ovaries, usually by direct extension of the inflammatory process from the bowel.[41] The presentation may be that of a unilateral adnexal mass. The diagnosis can be made via computed tomography (CT) scan, which would demonstrate a thickened abnormal ileum, and barium contrast studies will demonstrate primary bowel pathology. Recent advances in immunotherapy have seen many inhibitors of proinflammatory cytokines being introduced into the treatment of inflammatory bowel disease, especially the inhibitors to TNF-(alpha symbol) such as Infliximab. However, TNF-(alpha symbol) inhibitors are very expensive and have also been associated with multiple side effects such as severe infections, neurological events, hypersensitivities, and heart failure. Hence, these drugs are currently only used in cases of severe active Crohn's disease that is refractory to other forms of treatment.

Inflammation, Adhesion Formation, and Tubal Disease

One of the common consequences of pelvic infection is the formation of pelvic adhesions, where the fimbriae ends of the Fallopian tubes are obliterated and the ovaries adhere to the pelvic sidewall, which can result in pain and subfertility. Concurrent inflammation in the peritoneum because of infection causes peritonitis with the occurrence of severe pelvic and tubo-ovarian adhesions.

When the pelvis is inflamed, the mesothelial cells, which make up the peritoneum, secrete IL-1, 6, and 8, (TNF-α), transforming growth factor beta (TGF-β) tissue plasminogen activator and plasminogen activator inhibitors (PAI) and various other adhesion molecules.[42] As part of the healing process after the initial infective/inflammatory insult to the peritoneum, there is cellular infiltration and a growth response by the mesothelial cells in the damaged area. In response to the initial injury, resident cells in the peritoneum such as macrophages and mesothelial cells produce cellular mediators, which serve to modulate and orchestrate the subsequent response of the other cells involved in the inflammatory response. There is increased vascular permeability in vessels supplying the damaged area, followed by an exudation of inflammatory cells, ultimately leading to the formation of a fibrin matrix. The fibrin matrix is gradually organized and replaced by tissue containing fibroblasts, macrophages, and giant cells. This fibrin matrix connects two injured peritoneal surfaces forming fibrin bands. These fibrin bands can be broken down by fibrinolysis into smaller molecules as fibrin degradation products (FDP). Under conditions of aberrant peritoneal healing, ischemia results in a reduction in fibrinolytic activity and thus the persistence of the fibrin bands (Fig. 4.6). The organization of the fibrin bands over time results in the adhesions persisting. Clearly, the adhesion formation process also involves various other systems, mainly the interactions between the fibrinolytic system and other proteinases, particularly the metalloproteinases (MMPs) and their inhibitors – tissue inhibitors of metalloproteinases (TIMPs). MMPs and TIMPs are both important players in the remodeling of the extracellular matrix (ECM) (Fig. 4.7).

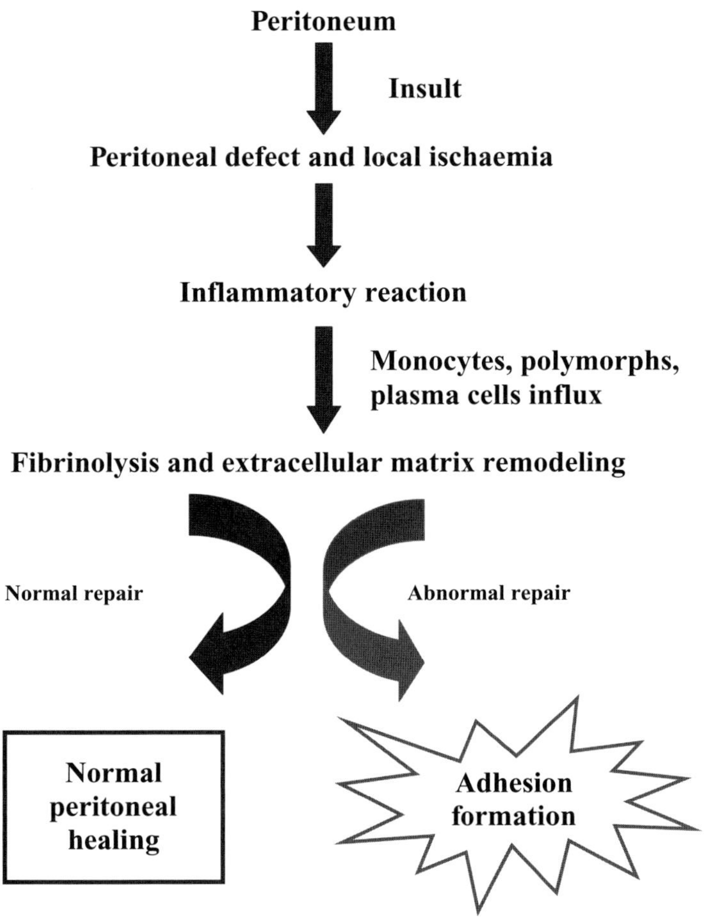

Fig. 4.6: A summary of normal tissue repair and adhesion formation following surgical trauma. After trauma to the peritoneum, an inflammatory reaction at the site of injury is evoked and the influx of the cellular components involved in inflammation occurs. Depending on the processes of inflammation, fibrinolysis, and extracellular matrix remodeling, normal or abnormal healing can result, the latter resulting in adhesion formation. (See Color Plate 5.)

Infection and inflammation of the Fallopian tubes therefore can result in intratubal pathology as well as extratubal adhesions, both of which simultaneously contribute to subfertility. There is evidence that the removal of the peritubal and periovarian adhesions can improve fertility,[43] although there is yet no effective prevention of adhesion reformation after their removal. Furthermore, intratubal mucosal damage, a consequence of many of these pelvic infections, is irreversible.

CONCLUSION

Infection and inflammatory conditions in the pelvis can lead to tubal disease and adhesion formation. A prime consideration for diagnostic workup to detect tubal pathology should be a *C. trachomatis* antibody test (or combination of tests as outlined in Table 4.1) and then proceed to HSSG, providing that the antibody levels are indicative of *C. trachomatis* infection. Anti-inflammatory drugs such as the nonsteroidals have not been shown to be effective in the prevention of adhesions once the infection and inflammation have begun. One of the possible reasons for this may be that they lack specificity. Clearly, there is value in screening programs to detect more important infections such as *C. trachomatis* where

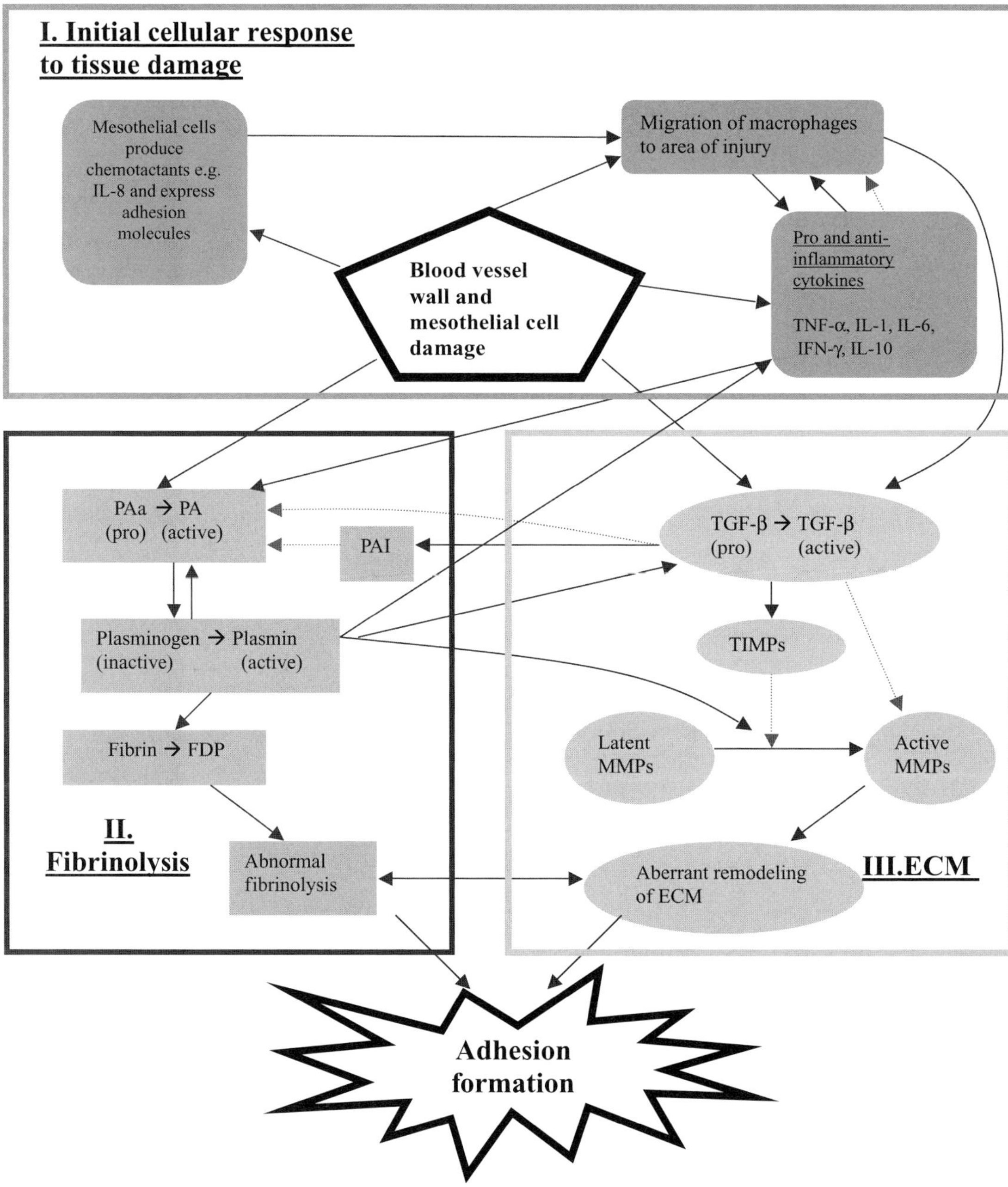

Fig. 4.7: A summary of three important pathways leading to adhesion formation: (I) initial cellular response to tissue damage (green); (II) fibrinolysis (blue); and (III) components of ECM (yellow). Blue bold arrows: stimulatory effect; red dotted arrows: inhibitory effect. For clarity of the figure, functions of the components considered important in adhesion formation are illustrated. Legend: ECM: Extracellular Matrix, MMP: Matrix metalloproteinase, TIMP: Tissue inhibitor of metalloproteinase. (See Color Plate 6.)

prevalence rates are high; however, this does not apply to other infectious causes of tubal damage. One strategy that has yet to be explored as part of a subfertility workup is to quantify levels of proinflammatory markers such as certain cytokines found in the genital tract secretions as early markers of possible tubal disease.

REFERENCES

1. Taraktchoglou M et al. Infectivity of Chlamydia trachomatis serovar LGV but not E is dependent on host cell heparan sulfate. *Infect Immun.* 2001;**69**(2):968–76.
2. Stephens RS, Poteralski JM, Olinger L. Interaction of Chlamydia trachomatis with mammalian cells is independent of host cell surface heparan sulfate glycosaminoglycans. *Infect Immun.* 2006;**74**(3):1795–9.
3. Gerbase AC et al. Global prevalence and incidence estimates of selected curable STDs. *Sex Transm Infect.* 1998;**74 Suppl 1**:S12–16.
4. Eley A et al. Prevalence of Chlamydia trachomatis IgG antibodies in antenatal patients from Trinidad. *Sex Transm Infect.* 2001;**77**(4):301–2.
5. Barlow RE et al. The prevalence of Chlamydia trachomatis in fresh tissue specimens from patients with ectopic pregnancy or tubal factor infertility as determined by PCR and in-situ hybridisation. *J Med Microbiol.* 2001;**50**(10):902–8.
6. Keay SD et al. The relation between immunoglobulin G antibodies to Chlamydia trachomatis and poor ovarian response to gonadotropin stimulation before in vitro fertilization. *Fertil Steril.* 1998;**70**(2):214–18.
7. Centers on Disease Control and Prevention (CDC). *Sexually transmitted disease surveillance.* Atlanta, GA: U.S. Department of Health and Human Services, 2000.
8. Catchpole M, Robinson A, Temple A. Chlamydia screening in the United Kingdom. *Sex Transm Infect.* 2003;**79**(1):3–4.
9. Westrom LV. Chlamydia and its effect on reproduction. *J Br Fer Soc.* 1996;**1**(1):23–30.
10. Kinnunen A et al. Chlamydial heat shock protein 60–specific T cells in inflamed salpingeal tissue. *Fertil Steril.* 2002;**77**(1):162–6.
11. Patton DL et al. The effects of Chlamydia trachomatis on the female reproductive tract of the Macaca nemestrina after a single tubal challenge following repeated cervical inoculations. *Obstet Gynecol.* 1990;**76**(4):643–50.
12. van Valkengoed IG et al. Overestimation of complication rates in evaluations of Chlamydia trachomatis screening programmes – implications for cost-effectiveness analyses. *Int J Epidemiol.* 2004;**33**(2):416–25.
13. Centers for Disease Control and Prevention. *Sexually transmitted disease surveillance.* Atlanta, GA: U.S. Department of Health and Human Services, 2002.
14. Tiitinen A et al. Chlamydia trachomatis and chlamydial heat shock protein 60-specific antibody and cell-mediated responses predict tubal factor infertility. *Hum Reprod.* 2006;**21**(6):1533–8.
15. Rank RG, Sanders MM, Patton DL. Increased incidence of oviduct pathology in the guinea pig after repeat vaginal inoculation with the chlamydial agent of guinea pig inclusion conjunctivitis. *Sex Transm Dis.* 1995;**22**(1):48–54.
16. Kimani J et al. Risk factors for Chlamydia trachomatis pelvic inflammatory disease among sex workers in Nairobi, Kenya. *J Infect Dis.* 1996;**173**(6):1437–44.
17. Cohen CR et al. Human leukocyte antigen class II DQ alleles associated with Chlamydia trachomatis tubal infertility. *Obstet Gynecol.* 2000;**95**(1):72–7.
18. Kinnunen AH et al. HLA DQ alleles and interleukin-10 polymorphism associated with Chlamydia trachomatis-related tubal factor infertility: a case-control study. *Hum Reprod.* 2002;**17**(8):2073–8.
19. Barr EL et al. Host inflammatory response and development of complications of Chlamydia trachomatis genital infection in CCR5-deficient mice and subfertile

women with the CCR5delta32 gene deletion. *J Microbiol Immunol Infect.* 2005;**38**(4): 244–54.

20. Morre SA et al. The role that the functional Asp299Gly polymorphism in the toll-like receptor-4 gene plays in susceptibility to Chlamydia trachomatis-associated tubal infertility. *J Infect Dis.* 2003;**187**(2):341–2; author reply 342–3.
21. Read R, Dower S, Eley A. Response to "The role that the functional Asp229 Gly polymorphism in the toll-like receptor 4 gene plays in susceptibility to Chlamydia trachomatis-associated tubal infertility." *J Infect Dis.* 2003;**187**:341–3.
22. Dean D, Suchland RJ, Stamm WE. Evidence for long-term cervical persistence of Chlamydia trachomatis by omp1 genotyping. *J Infect Dis.* 2000;**182**(3):909–16.
23. Carlson JH et al. Polymorphisms in the Chlamydia trachomatis cytotoxin locus associated with ocular and genital isolates. *Infect Immun.* 2004;**72**(12):7063–72.
24. Murillo LS et al. Interleukin-1B (IL-1B) and interleukin-1 receptor antagonist (IL-1RN) gene polymorphisms are not associated with tubal pathology and Chlamydia trachomatis-related tubal factor subfertility. *Hum Reprod.* 2003;**18**(11):2309–14.
25. Mpiga P et al. Sustained interleukin-6 and interleukin-8 expression following infection with Chlamydia trachomatis serovar L2 in a HeLa/THP-1 cell co-culture model. *Scand J Immunol.* 2006;**63**(3):199–207.
26. Gerard HC et al. Synovial Chlamydia trachomatis in patients with reactive arthritis/Reiter's syndrome are viable but show aberrant gene expression. *J Rheumatol.* 1998;**25**(4):734–42.
27. den Hartog JE et al. Serological markers of persistent C. trachomatis infections in women with tubal factor subfertility. *Hum Reprod.* 2005;**20**(4):986–90.
28. Dadamessi I, Eb F, Betsou F. Combined detection of Chlamydia trachomatis-specific antibodies against the 10 and 60-kDa heat shock proteins as a diagnostic tool for tubal factor infertility: Results from a case-control study in Cameroon. *FEMS Immunol Med Microbiol.* 2005;**45**(1):31–5.
29. Logan S et al. Can history, ultrasound, or ELISA chlamydial antibodies, alone or in combination, predict tubal factor infertility in subfertile women? *Hum Reprod.* 2003;**18**(11):2350–6.
30. Minassian SS, Wu CH. Chlamydia antibody by enzyme-linked immunosorbent assay and associated severity of tubal factor infertility. *Fertil Steril.* 1992;**58**(6):1245–7.
31. Witkin SS et al. Individual immunity and susceptibility to female genital tract infection. *Am J Obstet Gynecol.* 2000;**183**(1):252–6.
32. Debattista J et al. Immunopathogenesis of Chlamydia trachomatis infections in women. *Fertil Steril.* 2003;**79**(6):1273–87.
33. Simms I, Stephenson JM. Pelvic inflammatory disease epidemiology: what do we know and what do we need to know? *Sex Transm Infect.* 2000;**76**(2):80–7.
34. Meyer L et al. Surveillance of sexually transmitted diseases in France: recent trends and incidence. *Genitourin Med.* 1994;**70**(1):15–21.
35. Bevan CD et al. Clinical, laparoscopic, and microbiological findings in acute salpingitis: report on a United Kingdom cohort. *Br J Obstet Gynaecol.* 1995;**102**(5):407–14.
36. Edwards JL, Apicella MA. The molecular mechanisms used by Neisseria gonorrhoeae to initiate infection differ between men and women. *Clin Microbiol Rev.* 2004;**17**(4):965–81, table of contents.
37. Maisey K et al. Expression of proinflammatory cytokines and receptors by human Fallopian tubes in organ culture following challenge with Neisseria gonorrhoeae. *Infect Immun.* 2003;**71**(1):527–32.
38. Tartaglia LA et al. A novel domain within the 55 kd TNF receptor signals cell death. *Cell.* 1993;**74**(5):845–53.
39. Ness RB et al. Associations among human leukocyte antigen (HLA) class II DQ variants, bacterial sexually transmitted diseases, endometritis, and fertility among women with clinical pelvic inflammatory disease. *Sex Transm Dis.* 2004;**31**(5):301–4.
40. Schaefer G. Female genital tuberculosis. *Clin Obstet Gynecol.* 1976;**19**(1):223–39.

41. Wlodarski FM, Trainer TD. Granulomatous oophoritis and salpingitis associated with Crohn's disease of the appendix. *Am J Obstet Gynecol.* 1975;**122**(4):527–8.
42. Cheong YC et al. Peritoneal healing and adhesion formation/reformation. *Hum Reprod Update.* 2001;**7**(6): 556–66.
43. Tulandi T, Falcone T, KafkaI. Second-look operative laparoscopy 1 year following reproductive surgery. *Fertil Steril.* 1989;**52**(3):421–4.
44. Mouton JW et al. Tubal factor pathology caused by Chlamydia trachomatis: the role of serology. *Int J STD AIDS.* 2002;**13 Suppl 2**:26–9.
45. Persson K et al. Antibodies to Chlamydia trachomatis heat shock proteins in women with tubal factor infertility are associated with prior infection by C. trachomatis but not by C. pneumoniae. *Hum Reprod.* 1999;**14**(8):1969–73.

V

MANAGEMENT OF PROXIMAL TUBAL OCCLUSION

Nadia Kabli and Togas Tulandi

Tubal occlusion accounts for 12 to 33 percent of infertility.[1] It could be divided into proximal, midtubal, and distal occlusion. Midtubal occlusion is usually iatrogenic because of tubal sterilization, and distal tubal occlusion is related to salpingitis.

There are two types of proximal tubal occlusions. True occlusion can be due to salpingitis, endometriosis, or rarely congenital malformation. Another type is apparent proximal occlusion that is due to tubal spasm at the time of hysterosalpingography. True proximal tubal occlusion (PTO) is one of the common indications for in vitro fertilization.

ANATOMY AND HISTOPATHOLOGY

The length of the intramural portion of the fallopian tube is 1 to 3.5 cm.[2] This part of the tube is under the influence of cyclic changes of estrogen and progesterone. In the follicular phase, estrogen stimulates the muscular layer of the tube to undergo spasm, and the cilia beat less frequently than after ovulation. In the secretory phase, progesterone relaxes the muscularis and the cilia beat more often toward the direction of uterine cavity. This facilitates transfer of fertilized oocyte into the uterine cavity.[3]

False Diagnosis

One should interpret hysterosalpingographic (HSG) findings of PTO with caution (Fig. 5.1). False diagnosis of PTO was reported in 26.5 to 50 percent of cases.[4] Presumably, this is because of tubal spasm that occurs as physiologic response to uterine distention or pain during the procedure.

Histopathologic analysis of the resected tubes from women with PTO diagnosed by hysterosalpingography and/or laparoscopy showed a variety of findings including normal (20% of the tubes), amorphous debris or adhesions (40%), and extensive fibrosis or salpingitis isthmica nodosa (about 40%).[5] In addition, we often find a combination of proximal and distal tubal occlusion (bipolar tubal occlusion).

One-third of the cases had amorphous casts in the lumen of the intramural tubes.[5] Organized and calcified tubal secretion forms the cast and occludes the tubal lumen. During HSG or during tubal cannulation, we frequently find a polyp in the lumen of proximal tube. However, it rarely causes complete tubal blockage.[3]

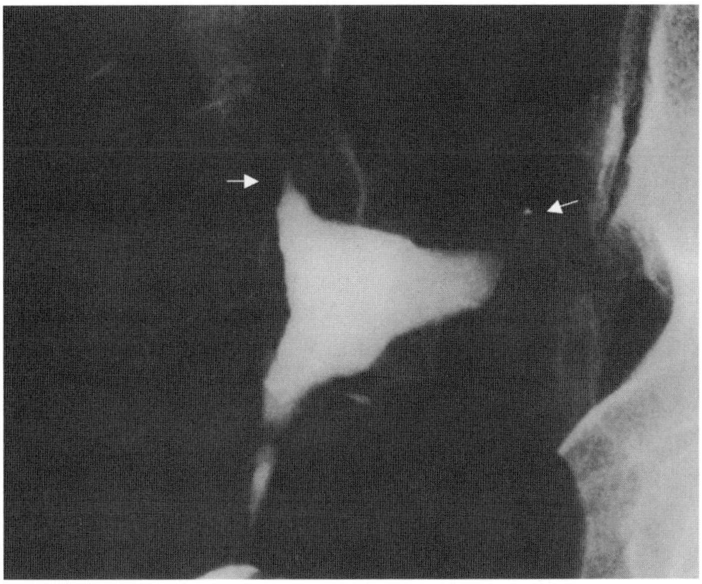

Fig. 5.1: Hysterosalpingographic findings of apparent proximal tubal occlusion.

True Occlusion

True cornual occlusion is usually due to salpingitis isthmica nodosa (SIN), where a firm nodule occludes and replaces the normal tissue in the cornual part of the tube. It accounts for 23 to 60 percent of histologically documented cases.[5] Grossly, the proximal tube is nodular and it has a firm consistency. The tubes are initially patent, but they become occluded with time[6] (Fig. 5.2). Besides infertility, SIN is associated with ectopic pregnancy.

The exact etiology of SIN is unclear. It could be congenital or related to a previous infection.[4–6] At hysterosalpingography (HSG), the radiologic contrast collects in diverticula that extend from the lumen of the intramural or isthmic portion of the tube.

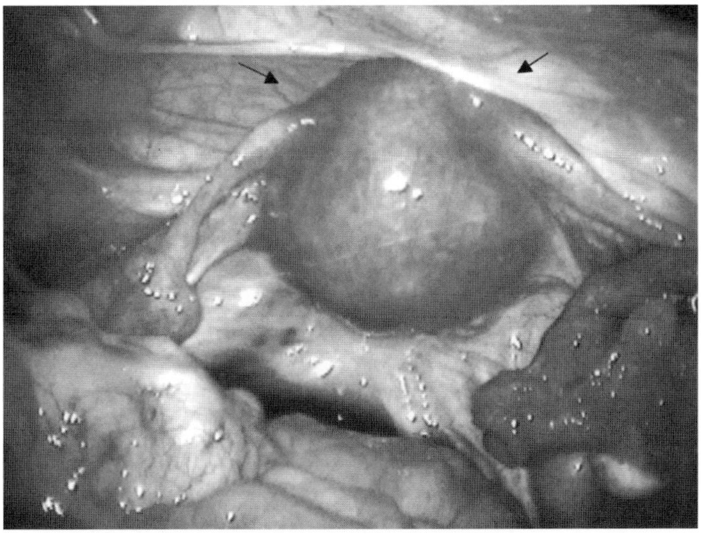

Fig. 5.2: Laparoscopic findings of salpingitis isthmica nodosa. (See Color Plate 7.)

Pelvic inflammatory disease (PID) is the most common cause of tubal factor infertility. In most cases, it involves the whole length of the tube resulting in peri-adnexal adhesions and hydrosalpinx. Recurrent PID occasionally causes isolated PTO.[5]

Endometriosis in the intramural portion of the tube is found in 7 to 14 percent of women with tubal factor infertility. The cyclic swelling of endometriosis deposits in the tubal wall results in progressive closure of the proximal tubal lumen.[7]

DIAGNOSTIC TESTS

Among different tests to evaluate tubal patency, hysterosalpingography remains the most widely used test. The presence of chlamydia antibody might raise a suspicion of tubal pathology. However, it is not specific for PTO.

Hysterosalpingography and Selective Tubal Catheterization

The high incidence of tubal spasm during hysterosalpingography is also illustrated by Desolle et al.[8] They performed a repeat HSG in forty women with radiologic findings of unilateral or bilateral PTO 1 month after the first, and found that twenty-four women had bilateral tubal patency.[8]

HSG is an important tool in the management of infertility. It provides information about the uterine cavity and the Fallopian tubes, and it facilitates spontaneous pregnancy. Spring et al.[9] evaluated the therapeutic effect of hysterosalpingography in 666 women with infertility. In their prospective randomized trial, the spontaneous conception rate was 30.6 percent within 1 year of the procedure, whereas the live birthrate in this cohort was 20.4 percent.[9]

Similar to hysterosalpingography, hysterosalpingo-contrast sonography (Hy-Co-Sy) is a procedure that evaluate the uterine cavity and the tubal patency, but under real-time ultrasound. It involves transcervical instillation of echogenic medium (air with saline or air-filled albumin microspheres). The accuracy of Hy-Co-Sy is comparable to that of HSG, but it is more costly.

Another diagnostic and possibly therapeutic technique is selective tubal catheterization (STC) or transcervical tubal cannulation.[5] STC is done using balloon angiographic catheters, or guidewires under fluoroscopic, hysteroscopic, or ultrasound guidance. In a study of seventy-two patients with true PTO,[4] canalization was successful for both tubes and for one tube in 34.7 percent and 61 percent of cases, respectively.

Laparoscopy

In women with hysterosalpingographic findings of PTO, chromopertubation during laparoscopy often reveals patent tubes. In the presence of SIN, the proximal tube is firm and nodular. Laparoscopy also allows evaluation of the entire tube, the presence of adhesions, and endometriosis.[4]

However, laparoscopy is no longer a routine diagnostic test for infertility. It is invasive and unnecessary for those undergoing in vitro fertilization (IVF) treatment. Our group perform diagnostic laparoscopy only in young women with possible tubal factor, endometriosis, or adnexal mass, who wish to be treated with non-IVF measures. In women older than age 35, we recommend IVF treatment.

MANAGEMENT

The treatment options for PTO depend on several factors including age, ovarian reserve, other infertility causes, and socioeconomic considerations. In order to eliminate false diagnosis, selective tubal catheterization should follow a radiological diagnosis of PTO.

Medical Approach

Because of the possibility of endometriosis-related PTO, a few authors have investigated the use of hormonal suppression. Muneyyirci-Delale et al. evaluated the effects of 3-month treatment with gonadotropin-releasing hormone agonist (GnRHa), norethindrone acetate, or danazol in twenty-three infertile women with PTO.[7] Following the treatment, sixteen of the twenty-three patients (69.6%) had at least one patent Fallopian tube, and nine patients conceived (39.1%).

In another small series of twenty-one patients, the authors confirmed the benefits of GnRHa in women with PTO.[10] They postulated that isolated proximal tubal blockage could be an estrogen-sensitive phenomenon. GnRHa increases the tubal patency and could increase conception rate.[10] Whether these patients had had true PTO is unknown. In addition, it is unclear how long the tubes would remain patent after discontinuation of GnRHa.

Radiologic Approach

In selective tubal catheterization or selective salpingography, injection of contrast medium can flush the proximal tube from debris creating a clear passage. If the tube remains occluded, further catheterization using a guidewire is followed. Tubal patency could be established, but the occlusion rate is high (30%) and there is a risk of tubal perforation (3–11%). This perforation usually heals spontaneously, but it may lead to intratubal adhesions and tubal dysfunction.

Al-Jaroudi et al. reported that among those with true occlusion, selective tubal catheterization results in a cumulative probability of conception of 28 percent, 59 percent, and 73 percent at 12-, 18-, and 24-month followup, respectively.[4] The median procedure-conception interval was 16.2 months. In another series of 218 patients with confirmed PTO, the spontaneous pregnancy rate 12 months after tubal catheterization was 47.2 percent.[3]

Inagaki et al. performed selective salpingography using hysteroscopic guidance[11] in forty-seven patients with unilateral or bilateral PTO. Twenty-seven patients (79.4%) with unilateral occlusion diagnosed by HSG were found to have normal patency by hysteroscopic selective salpingography. In patients with bilateral occlusion, 53.8 percent of patients had normal and patent tubes. The reason to perform the procedure in women with one patent tube is unclear.

In our experience what this means is selective filling of unilateral tube is a common occurrence at HSG and at chromopertubation during laparoscopy. Repeat tests would reveal that the tubes are patent; furthermore, the pregnancy rate with one or both tubes is similar.

Another technique is balloon tuboplasty. Using three different coronary angioplasty catheters, Osada et al. performed selective salpingography and balloon tuboplasty to treat PTO. The tubal patency rates ranged between 43 percent and 76 percent and the pregnancy rates were 30 to 52 percent.[12]

Surgical Approach

Before the development of in vitro fertilization (IVF), the only treatment for PTO was surgical reconstruction of the Fallopian tube. With the availability of IVF and nonsurgical treatments of PTO, today we rarely perform surgery for PTO. Occasionally we perform laparoscopic tubo-cornual anastomosis.

The traditional surgical treatment of PTO is uterotubal implantation. In this procedure, the intramural portion of the tube is resected, and a hole is drilled into the uterine cornua. The occluded part of the isthmic tube is incised repeatedly until the lumen is seen. The remaining distal part of the tube is inserted into the opening into the uterus and sutured (implantation).[13] Uterotubal implantation is associated with considerable bleeding and reocclusion tends to occur. In fact, tubal stenosis occurred in approximately 80 percent of cases. The pregnancy rate following this procedure is very low. This technique should be abandoned.

Unlike uterotubal implantation, with tubo-cornual anastomosis the cornual integrity is preserved. Indeed, the intramural portion of the tube is not usually occluded. The procedure is performed by incising the cornua repeatedly until a tubal opening is found. Tubo-cornual anastomosis is then performed.[13] We perform this procedure by laparoscopy (Fig. 5.3).

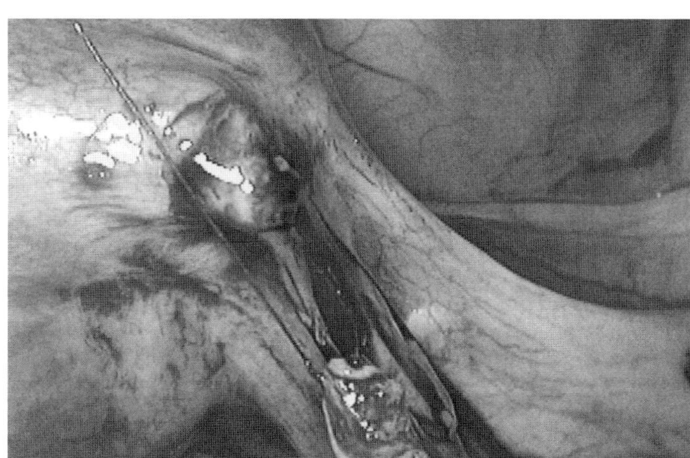

Fig. 5.3: Laparoscopic tubal anastomosis. (See Color Plate 8.)

Awartani and McComb reported the reproductive outcome after microsurgical resection and tubo-cornual anastomosis for the nonocclusive form of SIN in a small number of patients. They reported an intrauterine pregnancy rate of 46.1 percent and ectopic pregnancy of 11.6 percent at 12 months of followup. Whether these women would have a spontaneous conception without surgery is unknown. The study had no control group.[6]

Two meta-analyses revealed that the intrauterine pregnancy rate after microsurgical tubo-cornual anastomosis is superior to that after macrosurgical approach.[14,15] In any event, the results are inferior to those of IVF and the procedure requires a laparotomy incision. In addition, unlike IVF, pregnancy occurs many months after the surgery.

IN VITRO FERTILIZATION

IVF has become an almost universal treatment for infertility of any cause. It offers a pregnancy rate of approximately 25 to 30 percent and live birthrate of 20 percent per cycle.[16,17] These rates showed large variations among different institutions. The pregnancy rate was more than 35 percent in the United States, and the delivery rate per aspiration in North America was 30.6 percent.[17]

Unlike non-IVF treatments, the ectopic pregnancy rate with IVF is lower, and IVF does not carry the risks of surgery and general anesthesia. Today, there are no randomized trials comparing IVF versus tubal surgery in the treatment of women with tubal disease. The available evidence, however, argues against conducting such study.

Conclusions

PTO, suggested by failure of contrast medium to enter the intramural or isthmic portion of the tube, is diagnosed in 10 to 20 percent of hysterosalpingography. Due to the high incidence of false-positive results, a hysterosalpingographic finding of PTO must be followed by selective tubal catheterization. The cumulative pregnancy rate after tubal catheterization is 28 to 47 percent at 12 months followup. Approximately 20 percent of the tube could not be catheterized and the patients are best treated by IVF.

Surgical treatment of such a blockage is not highly successful. This is because of the severity of tubal damage, and in some cases, the distal tube is abnormal as well. There are two operative procedures to correct proximal tubal blockage: cornual reimplantation and tubo-cornual anastomosis. The pregnancy rate after tubo-cornual implantation is extremely low; this technique should be abandoned.

Tubo-cornual anastomosis is a better procedure; however, its place in the IVF era is limited. It can be offered to young women with true PTO who for some reason cannot be treated with IVF. Tubo-cornual anastomosis should be performed using microsurgical principles, preferably by laparoscopy. However, conception usually occurs many months after surgery and the incidence of ectopic pregnancy is high.

In this modern era of assisted reproductive technologies, reproductive surgery has a limited role for proximal tubal occlusion. PTO is best treated with IVF, especially in women over age 35 with a long history of infertility or those who require a laparotomy. Compared to non-IVF treatments, IVF leads to a low ectopic pregnancy rate and higher live birthrate in a short time.

REFERENCES

1. Catalano GF, Muzii L, Marana R. Tubal factor infertility. *Rays.* 1998;**23**:673–82.
2. Kerin JF, Surrey ES, Williams DB, Daykhovsky L, Grundfest WS. Falloposcopic observations of endotubal isthmic plugs as a cause of reversible obstruction and their histological characterization. *J Laparoendos Surg.* 1991;**1**:103–10.
3. Papaioannou S, Afnan M, Girling AJ, Coomarasamy A, Ola B, Olufowobi O, et al. Long-term fertility prognosis following selective salpingography and tubal catheterization in women with proximal tubal blockage. *Human Reprod.* 2002;**17**:2325–30.
4. Al-Jaroudi D, Herba MJ, Tulandi T. Reproductive performance after selective tubal catheterization. *J Min Inv Gynecol.* 2005;**12**:150–2.
5. Kodaman PH, Arici A, Seli E. Evidence-based diagnosis and management of tubal factor infertility. *Current Opinion Obstet Gynecol.* 2004;**16**:221–9.
6. Awartani K, McComb PF. Microsurgical resection of nonocclusive salpingitis isthmica nodosa is beneficial. *Fertil Steril.* 2003;**79**:1199–203.
7. Muneyyirci-Delale O, Karacan M. Hormonal treatment of bilateral proximal tubal obstruction. *Int J Fertil Womens Med.* 1999;**44**:204–8.
8. Dessole S, Meloni GB, Capobianco G, Manzoni MA, Ambrosini G, Canalis GC. A second hysterosalpingography reduces the use of selective technique for treatment of a proximal tubal obstruction. *Fertil Steril.* 2000;**73**:1037–9.
9. Spring DB BHPS. Potential therapeutic effects of contrast materials in hysterosalpingography: a prospective randomized clinical trial. *Kaiser Permanente Infertility Work Group. Radiol.* 2000;**214**:53–7.
10. Surrey ES, Bishop JA, Surrey MW. Role of GnRH agonists in managing proximal Fallopian tube obstruction. *J Reprod Med.* 2000;**45**:126–30.
11. Inagaki N, Sato K, Toyoshima K, et al. Hysteroscopic selective salpingography. *Fertil Steril.* 1999;**72**:733–6.
12. Osada H, Kiyoshi FT, Tsunoda I, Tsubata K, Satoh K, Palter SF. Outpatient evaluation and treatment of tubal obstruction with selective salpingography and balloon tuboplasty. *Fertil Steril.* 2000;**73**:1032–6.
13. Gomel V, McComb PF. Microsurgery for tubal infertility. *J Reprod Med.* 2006;**51**: 177–84.
14. Gomel V. Reproductive surgery. *Minerva Ginecologica.* 2005;**57**:21–8.
15. Ahmad G, Watson A, Vandekerckhove P, Lilford R. Techniques for pelvic surgery in subfertility. *Cochrane Database of Systematic Reviews.* 2006; Issue 2, CD000221. DOI. 10. 1002/14655818. CD 000221 Pub.**3**.
16. The European IVF-monitoring programme (EIM) for the European Society of Human Reproduction and Embryology (ESHRE), Andersen AN, Gianaroli L, Felberbaum R, de MJ, Nygren KG. Assisted reproductive technology in Europe, 2002. Results generated from European registers by ESHRE. *Human Reprod.* 2006;**21**:1680–97.
17. International Committee for Monitoring Assisted Reproductive Technology. Adamson GD, de Mouzon J, Lancaster P, Nygren KG, Sullivan E, Zegers-Hochschild F. World collaborative report on in vitro fertilization, 2000. *Fertil Steril.* 2006;**85**:1586–622.

VI

ECTOPIC PREGNANCY

Bassem Refaat and William L. Ledger

INTRODUCTION

Ectopic pregnancy (EP) is any pregnancy in which the fertilized ovum implants outside the intrauterine cavity. More than 95 percent of ectopic pregnancies occur in the Fallopian tubes (tubal pregnancy), mainly in the ampullary region. However, other parts of the tube are affected such as the isthmic or interstitial regions. Another 2.5 percent occur in the cornua of the uterus, and the remainder are found in the ovary, cervix, or abdominal cavity.[1] EP is an increasing health risk for women throughout the world and continues to be the leading cause of maternal death in the first trimester.[2,3] Although the incidence of ectopic pregnancy has been increasing in the last two decades, the combination of serum quantitative human chorionic gonadotrophin (hCG), transvaginal ultrasound, and laparoscopy have resulted in earlier diagnosis and treatment. In the UK, the incidence doubled from 4.9 to 9.6 per 1,000 pregnancies between 1973 and 1993, while mortality decreased from 16 to 3 per 10,000 cases of ectopic pregnancy.[4,5]

PATHOPHYSIOLOGY

The Fallopian tube plays an important role in transport and nutritional support of the gametes. Normally, an ovum is fertilized in the Fallopian tube and then travels down the tube to the intrauterine cavity for implantation. Through the actions of the smooth muscular layers and ciliated epithelium, the oocyte and then the zygote are transported to the endometrial cavity at the proper time for implantation. Any mechanism that interferes with the normal function of the Fallopian tube during this process increases the risk of ectopic pregnancy. Compromised tubal function can occur after external or internal injury. The mechanism can be anatomical (scars, adhesions, etc.) or functional (e.g., impaired tubal mobility).

RISK FACTORS

Controversy still surrounds the exact etiology of ectopic pregnancy; however, it contributes to poor reproductive performance among women of childbearing age.[6] Although a proportion of women with ectopic pregnancy have no identifiable causal factors, several factors increase the risk of ectopic pregnancy. These

Table 6.1 Risk Factors for Ectopic Pregnancy

A. Common risk factors
- Pelvic inflammatory disease (PID)
- Previous ectopic pregnancy
- Tubal surgery
- Sterilization and IUDs
- History of infertility
- IVF and embryo transfer
- Endometriosis
- Smoking
- Congenital uterotubal anomalies
- History of in utero exposure to diethylstilbestrol (DES)

B. Other risk factors
- Multiple sexual partners
- Early age at first intercourse
- Vaginal douching

factors share a common mechanism of action, namely interference with Fallopian tube function.[7] The most common risk factors associated with ectopic pregnancy are summarized in Table 6.1.

Pelvic Inflammatory Disease

In the general population, pelvic inflammatory disease (PID) is the most common risk factor associated with ectopic pregnancy.[8] A history of PID is particularly important and has been implicated in the increased incidence of EP.[9–11]

Organisms that preferentially attack the Fallopian tubes include *Neisseria gonorrhoeae*, *Chlamydia trachomatis*, and mixed aerobes and anaerobes. The most common causative organism of PID in the UK is *C. trachomatis*.[12,13]

Unlike mixed aerobes and anaerobes, *N. gonorrhoeae* and *C. trachomatis* can produce silent infections. *C. trachomatis* infection is the most common sexually transmitted infection throughout the world. The highest incidence of Chlamydia is in teens and young adults from ages 15 to 25. Chlamydia is a small intracellular bacterium that needs living cells to multiply. There are eighteen distinct serotypes of *C. trachomatis*, with serotypes D through K causing sexually transmitted genital infections and neonatal infection. *C. trachomatis* is the most important cause of mucopurulent cervicitis in women. Chlamydial cervicitis is usually asymptomatic and may be associated with ascending infection to the upper genital tract resulting in PID. Women are especially at risk for such consequence, because ascending Chlamydial infection can result in colonization of the endometrium and Fallopian tube epithelial cells. The immune response to this infection results in tubal occlusion, ectopic pregnancy, and infertility. A study has showed that the majority of the Fallopian tube biopsies collected at the time of salpingectomy expressed Chlamydial DNA by polymerase chain reaction (PCR). In addition, they suggested that the Chlamydial cells identified in the PCR were viable and metabolically active at the time of tissue biopsy. Another study suggested that Chlamydial DNA can persist in tissue specimens when

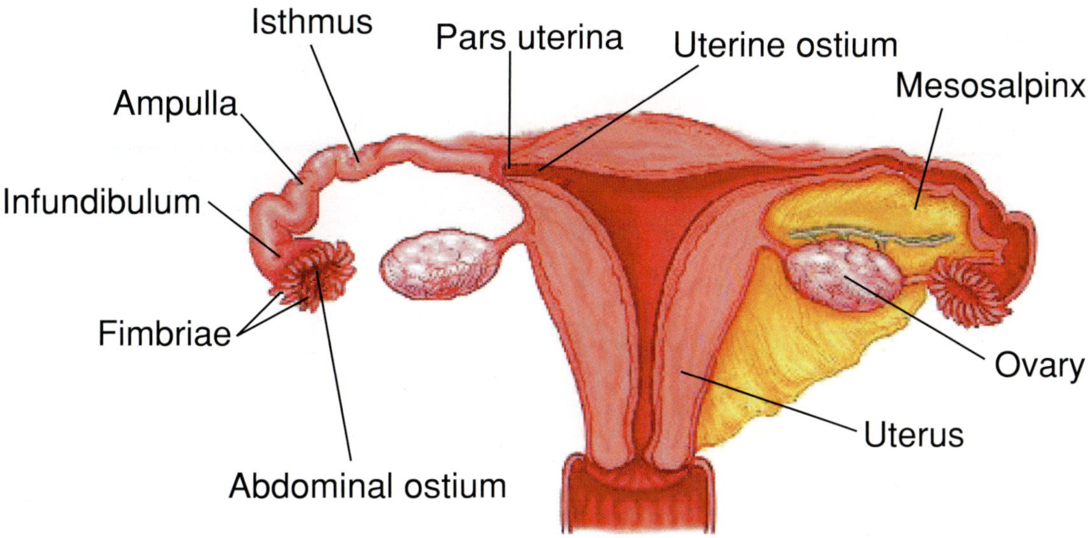

Plate 1: Anatomy of the Fallopian tubes.

Plate 2: Diagram of Fallopian tube showing different parts in cross-section: the proximal region (a) isthmus, the middle region (b) ampulla and the distal region, and (c) infundibulum.

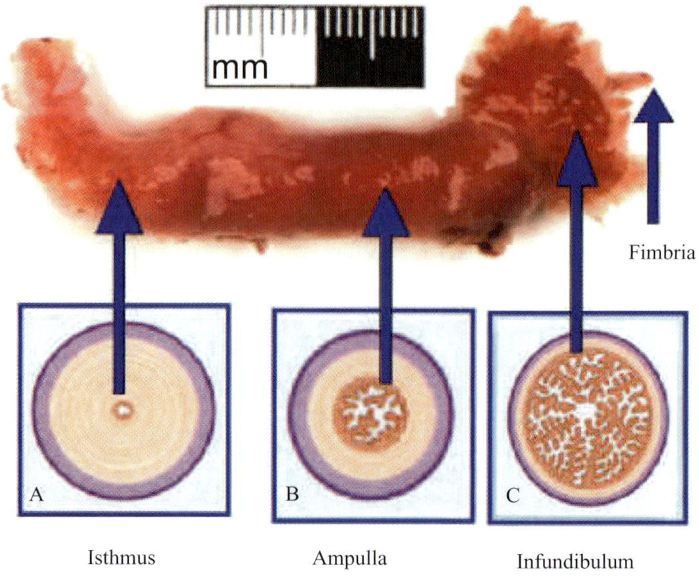

Plate 3: ELISA showing detection of chlamydial antibodies on a microtitre plate.

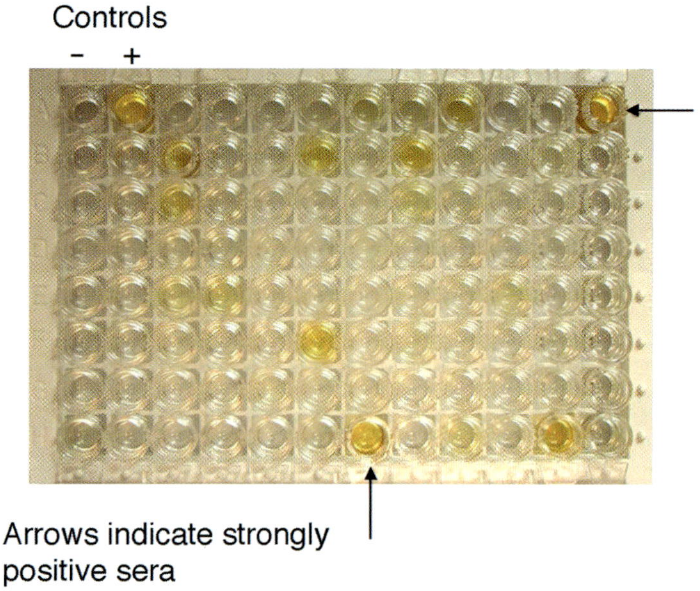

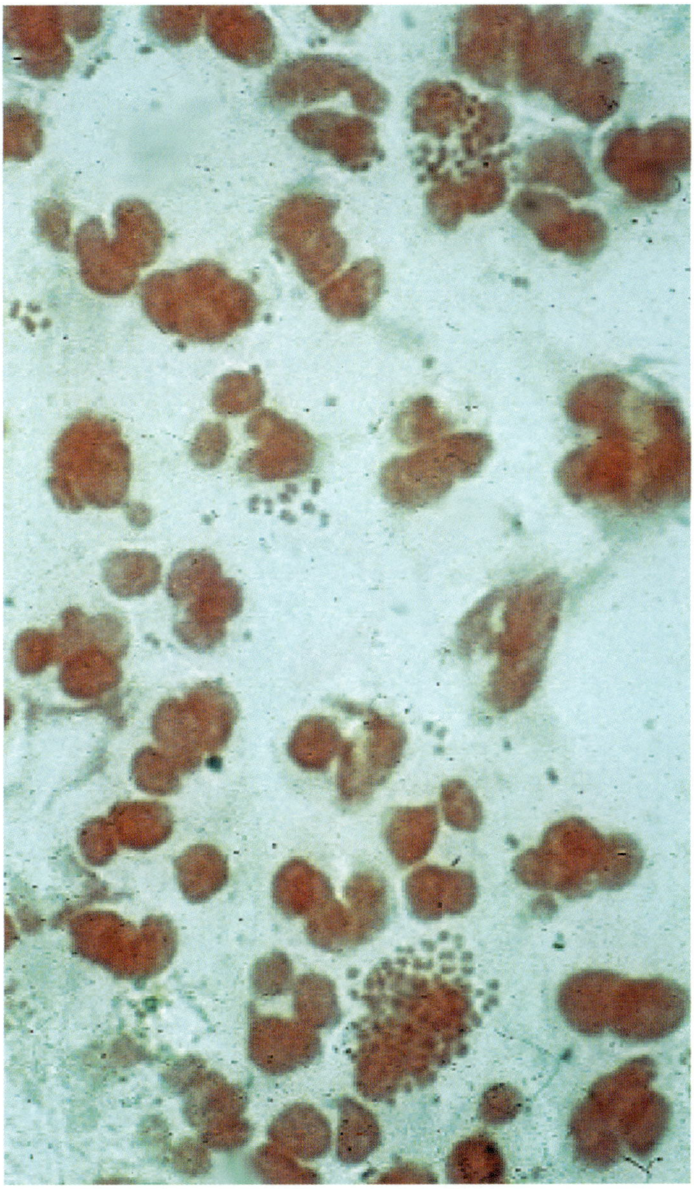

Plate 4: Gram stain of *Neisseria gonorrhoeae.*

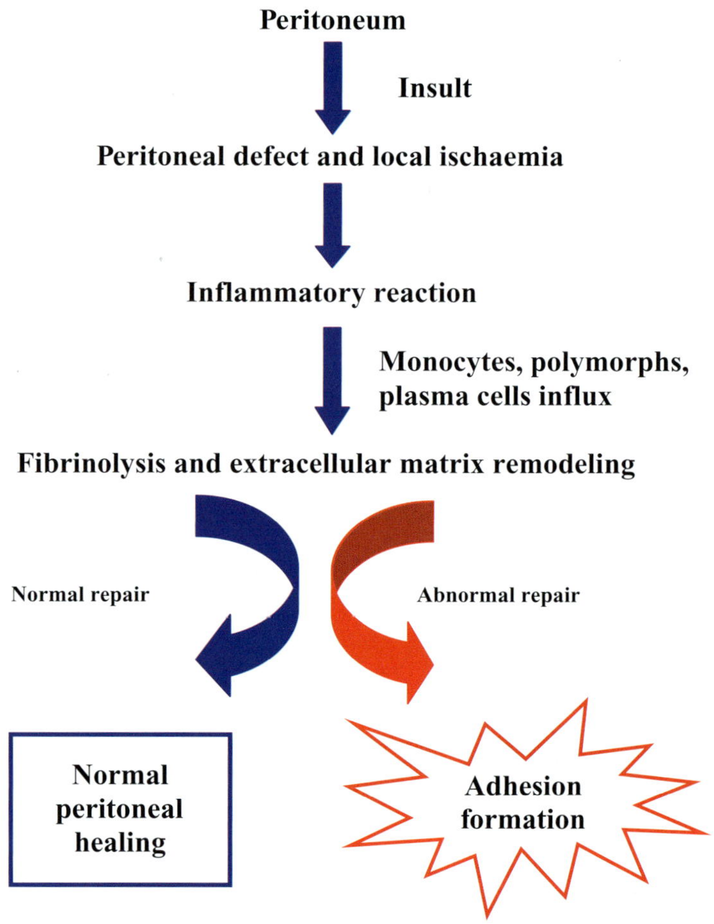

Plate 5: A summary of normal tissue repair and adhesion formation following surgical trauma. After trauma to the peritoneum, an inflammatory reaction at the site of injury is evoked and the influx of the cellular components involved in inflammation occurs. Depending on the processes of inflammation, fibrinolysis, and extracellular matrix remodeling, normal or abnormal healing can result, the latter resulting in adhesion formation.

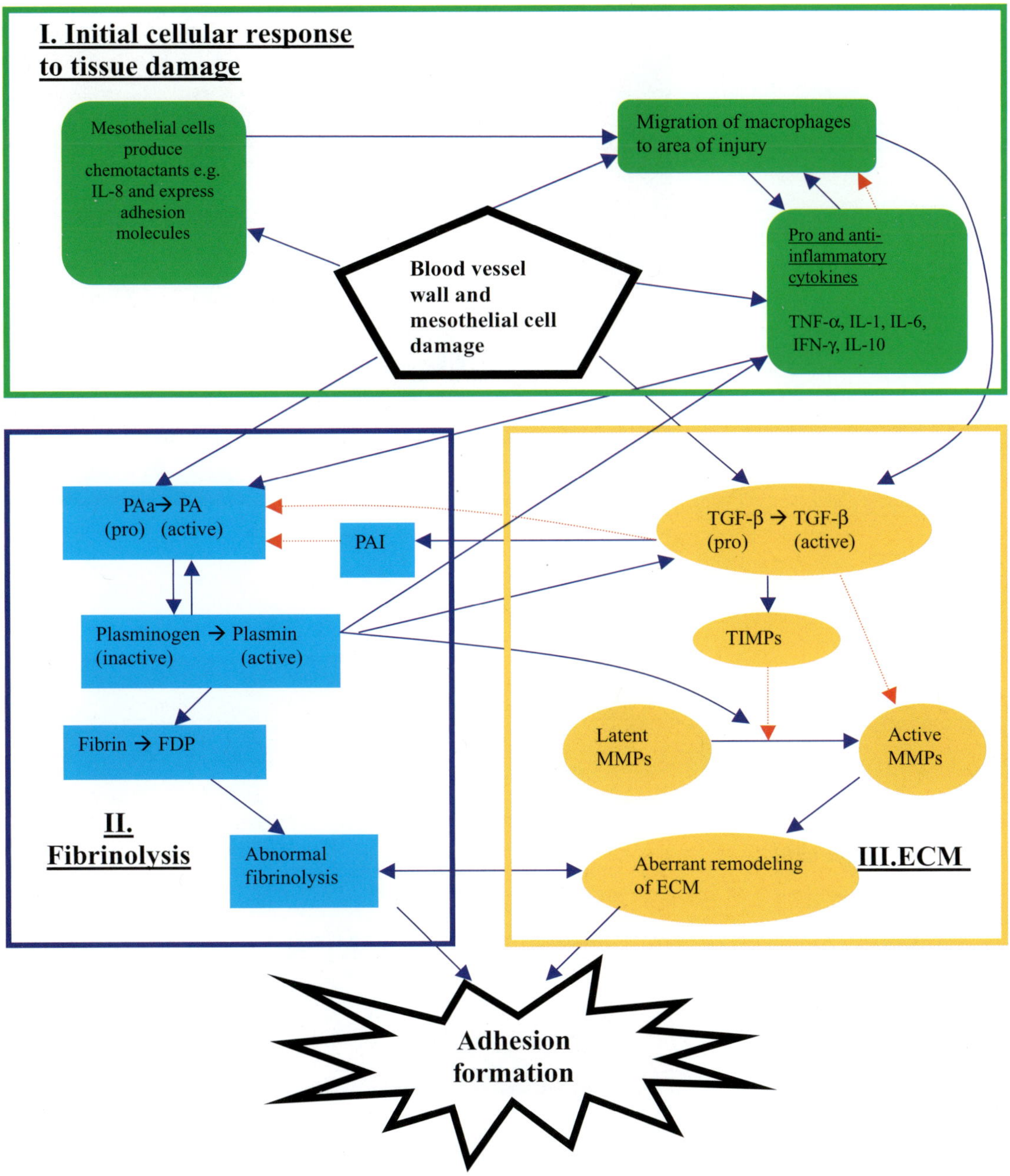

Plate 6: A summary of three important pathways leading to adhesion formation: (I) initial cellular response to tissue damage (green); (II) fibrinolysis (blue); and (III) components of ECM (yellow). Blue bold arrows: stimulatory effect; red dotted arrows: inhibitory effect. For clarity of the figure, functions of the components considered important in adhesion formation are illustrated. Legend: ECM: Extracellular Matrix, MMP: Matrix metalloproteinase, TIMP: Tissue inhibitor of metalloproteinase.

Plate 7: Laparoscopic findings of salpingitis isthmica nodosa.

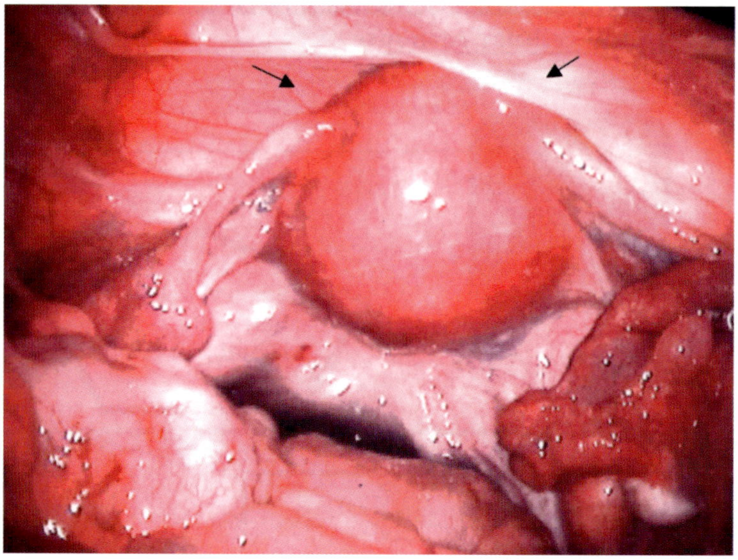

Plate 8: Laparoscopic tubal anastomosis.

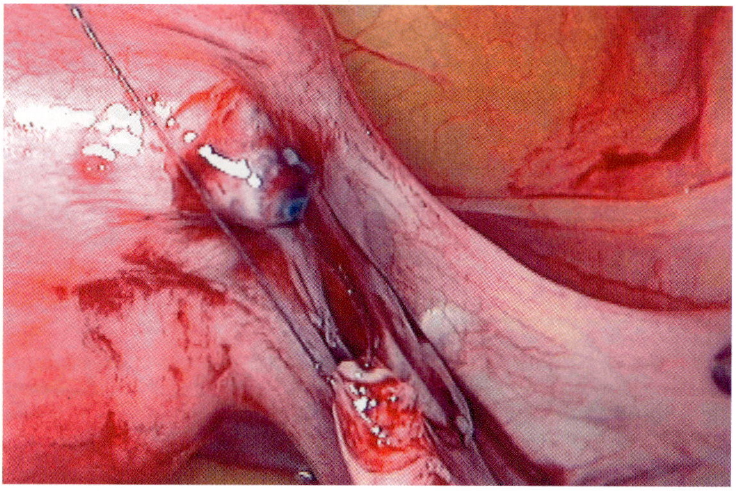

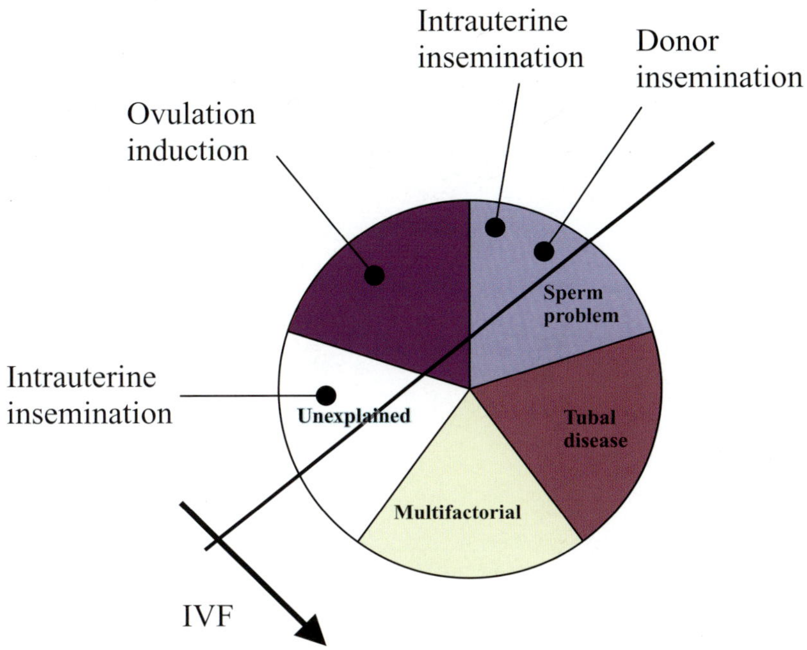

Plate 9: Treatments of choice for subfertility with different etiologies. The etiology of subfertility can be divided into five groups of roughly equal prevalence. IVF provides the highest chance of pregnancy for most subfertile couples and in particular for all those with tubal disease.

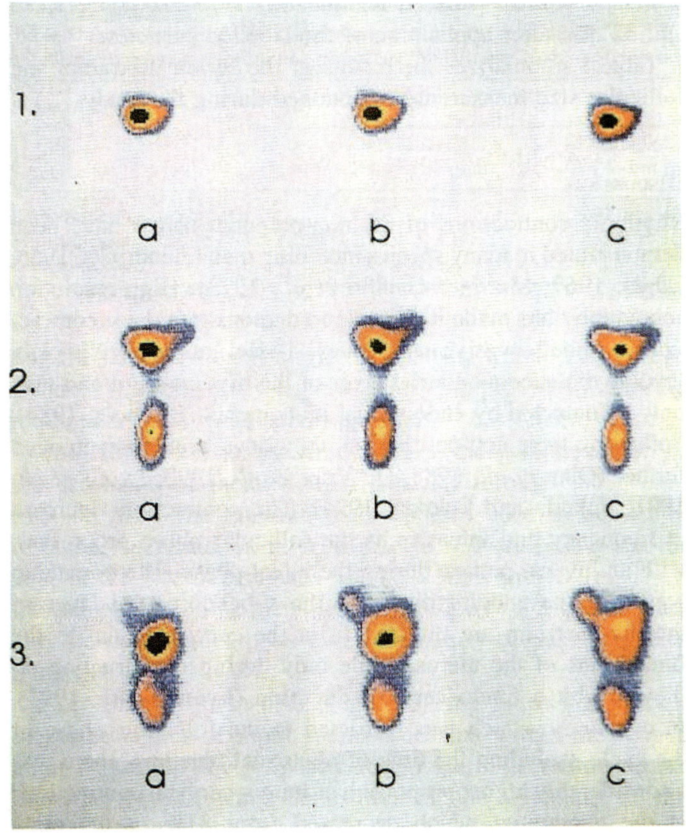

Plate 10: Hysterosalpingo Scintilography in three different patients (panel 1, early follicular phase; panel 2, mid-follicular phase; panel 3, late follicular phase). In each patient, scintigrams were performed at 1 minute (a), 16 minutes (b), and 32 minutes (c) after vaginal application of radioactive labeled macropheres. With permission from Kunz et al., *Human Reproduction* 1996, **11**:627–32.

the organism cannot otherwise be detected. The precise mechanism by which Chlamydial infection results in tubal damage is still unclear. In women infected with these organisms, even early treatment does not necessarily prevent tubal damage.[14,15] After acute salpingitis, the risk of an ectopic pregnancy is increased by sevenfold.[9] Comprehensive programs to prevent Chlamydia infection not only decrease the incidence of *C. trachomatis* infections, but also the rate of ectopic pregnancies.[16,17]

Previous Ectopic Pregnancy

Previous ectopic pregnancy becomes a more significant risk factor with each successive occurrence.[18] With one previous ectopic pregnancy treated by linear salpingostomy, the recurrence rate ranges from 15 to 20 percent, depending on the integrity of the contralateral tube.[1,19] Two previous ectopic pregnancies increase the risk of recurrence to 32 percent, although an intervening intrauterine pregnancy lowers this rate.[1,20]

Contraception and IUDs

Previous female sterilization[21] and current use of intrauterine devices (IUDs)[22] are only risk factors when comparing ectopic pregnancy with pregnant controls and not with nonpregnant controls. This is because overall the risk of pregnancy in these situations is low. However, if pregnancy occurs, an ectopic pregnancy is more likely. The risk of ectopic pregnancy after sterilization has been reported as 7.3 per 1,000 pregnancies within 10 years.[22]

IUDs may have an etiological role in EP.[23] One explanation for the perceived association of IUD use with ectopic pregnancy may be that when an IUD is present, ectopic pregnancy occurs more often than intrauterine pregnancy. Simply because IUDs are more effective in preventing intrauterine pregnancy than ectopic pregnancy, implantation is more likely to occur in an ectopic location.[1,24] Recent advances in intrauterine contraceptive technology have decreased IUD-induced EP. The levonorgestrel intrauterine system (LNG-IUS) is very effective in preventing intrauterine pregnancy and possibly ectopic pregnancy.[25] The rate of EP was significantly lower in users of LNG-IUS (e.g., Mirena) compared with those using copper-bearing IUDs.[26] However, if failure occurs, there may be a higher risk of tubal pregnancy.[27,28] Levonorgestrel-releasing implants (Implanon) are also highly effective contraceptives with low risk of EP.[29] It has been reported that progesterone downregulates LH-receptors, which is a regulatory factor for tubal contractility in porcine oviduct.[30] In addition, insulin-like growth factor binding protein-1 (IGFBP-1), which is a regulatory factor for implantation, is inhibited by progesterone.[31]

History of Infertility and IVF Treatment

Although in vitro fertilization (IVF)/embryo transfer was developed to bypass tubal factor infertility, increasing numbers of unusual forms of ectopic pregnancies are being reported after IVF/embryo transfer treatment.[32,33] Of all clinical pregnancies that occur with IVF, 4 percent are likely to be ectopic.[34,35] The majority of these are tubal ectopic pregnancies. This is two to three times greater than the background incidence. The main risk factor in this group is tubal infertility.[34,35] The incidence of heterotopic pregnancy (an ectopic pregnancy together with an intrauterine pregnancy) is also increased after assisted reproductive techniques.[36] A possible influence of embryo transfer technique in the etiology of ectopic pregnancy has been discussed.[37,38] They discussed the possible effect of the volume of culture media used at embryo transfer. Transfer of embryos in a small volume of culture media (10–20 ml) has been advised to prevent reflux into the Fallopian tube. It has also been proposed that transfer of embryos to a standard midcavity position results in a lower ectopic pregnancy rate.

Endometriosis

Several studies have reported an association between endometriosis and ectopic pregnancy.[20,39,40] Endometriosis results in pelvic and tubal adhesions and abnormal tubal function. The Fallopian tubes may also be affected by other, less clearly understood causes of infertility,[40] as well as many of the hormones that are administered to aid ovulation and improve fertility.[20]

Cigarette Smoking

Cigarette smoking has an independent and dose-related effect on the risk of ectopic pregnancy.[41] Smoking is known to affect ciliary action in the nasopharynx and respiratory tract. A similar effect may occur within the Fallopian tube[42,43] leading to tubal ciliary beat frequency and coordination impairment and development of ectopic pregnancy.

DES and Other Anatomical Effects

In utero exposure to diethylstilbestrol (DES) is associated with uterotubal anomalies ranging from gross structural abnormalities such as a double uterus to more subtle microscopic abnormalities resulting in tubal dysfunction. Any uterotubal anomalies (tubal hypoplasia, tortuosity, congenital diverticula, accessory ostia, partial stenosis), with or without DES exposure, increase the risk of ectopic pregnancy.[44]

Other Risk Factors

Multiple sexual partners, early age at first intercourse, and vaginal douching are often considered risk factors for ectopic pregnancy. The mechanism of action for these risk factors is indirect, in that they are markers for the development of sexually transmitted disease, ascending infection, or both.[20,42]

Table 6.2 Clinical Picture of Ectopic Pregnancy

A. Symptoms
- History of amenorrhea (6–8 weeks)
- Abdominal pain
- Vaginal bleeding
- Shoulder tip discomfort
- Pain on defecation/micturition
- Syncope and/or hypovolemic shock in acute cases

B. Signs
- Normal or slightly enlarged uterus
- Palpable adnexal mass
- Signs of intraperitoneal hemorrhage (rupture/leakage)
- Pain on movement of the cervix (cervical excitation)

CLINICAL PRESENTATION

Between 40 and 50 percent of ectopic pregnancies are misdiagnosed at the initial visit to an emergency department.[45,46] Failure to identify risk factors is cited as a common and significant reason for misdiagnosis.[45] A proper history and physical examination remain the foundation of initiating an appropriate workup that will result in the accurate and timely diagnosis of an ectopic pregnancy. Identification of risk factors can increase the index of suspicion and provide significance to minor physical findings (Table 6.2).

Symptoms

Historically, the hallmark of ectopic pregnancy has been a triad of a period of amenorrhea (6–8 weeks), abdominal pain, and vaginal bleeding. This remains the most common presentation of tubal pregnancy in symptomatic patients. Other presentations depend on the location of the ectopic pregnancy. Less commonly, ectopic pregnancy presents with pain radiating to the shoulder, syncope, and/or hypovolemic shock. Up to 9 percent of women with ectopic pregnancy report no pain and one-third lack adnexal tenderness. Although the presence of known risk factors – abdominal pain and vaginal bleeding after an interval of amenorrhea – increase suspicion, they are not sufficient to confirm or exclude a diagnosis of ectopic pregnancy.[3]

However, any sexually active woman presenting with abdominal pain and vaginal bleeding following a period of amenorrhea should be considered to have an ectopic pregnancy until proved otherwise. Therefore, if there is any suspicion, hospital referral for investigation is compulsory.

Signs

On examination, a normal or slightly enlarged uterus, a palpable adnexal mass, and signs of intraperitoneal hemorrhage, which include abdominal tenderness, peritonism, abdominal distention, or pain on movement of the cervix (cervical

Table 6.3 Summary of Investigations

A. Biochemical markers
- hCG
  - Detected in maternal serum within 7 days
  - It is 99% sensitive and specific for pregnancy
  - Provides supporting evidence in the diagnosis of EP
  - Combined with imaging results, it outlines the management of EP
- PAPP-A
  - Can distinguish between PF and normal IUP but not EP and abIUP
- Progesterone
  - Might be useful to differentiate between abIUP and EP
- Other hormones
  - Inhibin-A decreases by 40% in EP

B. Imaging
- Transvaginal ultrasound
  - Identifies gestational sac at serum hCG 1,000 to 1,500 IU/L
- Abdominal ultrasound
  - Identifies gestational sac at serum hCG 6,500 IU/L

C. Laparoscopy
- Was the first step in the diagnostic management of EP
- Remained the only reliable method for diagnosing of EP until the late 1980s

excitation), may be seen. Findings such as hypotension and marked abdominal tenderness with guarding and rebound tenderness suggest a leaking or ruptured ectopic pregnancy.

DIAGNOSIS

Although the incidence of ectopic pregnancy has been increasing in the past two decades, several diagnostic innovations have resulted in earlier diagnosis and treatment (Table 6.3).

Biochemical Markers

Human Chorionic Gonadotropin (hCG)

hCG is one of the earliest placental secretory products. Its function in early pregnancy is to "rescue" the corpus luteum and maintain uterine quiescence by promoting luteal secretion of progesterone. Following conception, hCG can be detected in maternal serum within 7 days and in maternal urine by the time the first period would have been due if conception had not occurred. After a careful history and physical examination, a standard pregnancy test may be performed by measuring urine beta-hCG level. A modern urinary pregnancy test is 99 percent sensitive and 99 percent specific for pregnancy.[47]

Although used as the initial step in some settings, the urine pregnancy test is a qualitative rather than quantitative measure that identifies the presence of hCG in concentrations as low as 25 IU/L. Measuring serum beta-hCG concentration is quantitative and provides better evidence in the diagnosis of ectopic pregnancy. In addition, the combination of serum beta-hCG concentrations with imaging techniques defines the process of diagnosis of ectopic pregnancy.

Pregnancy Associated Plasma Protein-A

Pregnancy associated plasma protein-A (PAPP-A), which is a macromolecular glycoprotein produced by the trophoblast, increases throughout pregnancy. Although PAPP-A has no identifiable biological function, several studies have investigated the clinical usefulness of its measurement during pregnancy. PAPP-A might be used as a marker for early pregnancy failure (PF) with sensitivity value of 54.2 percent and specificity value of 99 percent. However, it cannot distinguish between abnormal intrauterine pregnancy (abIUP) and ectopic pregnancy.[48]

Progesterone

A single progesterone measurement has the ability to distinguish between early pregnancy failure and normal intrauterine pregnancy (IUP). However, its usefulness to differentiate between abIUP and EP is subject to debate. Some studies showed that progesterone level was significantly decreased in abIUP compared to EP,[48] whereas a meta-analysis reported that a single progesterone measurement could not discriminate between abIUP and EP.[68]

Other Markers

Several studies have investigated a possible role for other molecules in the diagnosis of ectopic pregnancy. It has been reported that inhibin-A, a heterodimeric glycoprotein secreted by the placenta in early pregnancy, is decreased by 40 percent in EP compared to normal IUP.[50] However, at the present time, the most reliable marker for EP diagnosis is serum β-hCG measurement with specificity 99 percent and sensitivity 99 percent.[47]

Imaging Techniques

Ultrasound

Ultrasound can be used to locate a pregnancy anatomically and to see if the fetus is alive. In general, a gestational sac can be consistently identified by transvaginal ultrasound (TV) when the serum hCG level exceeds 1,000 to 1,500 IU/L.[51,52] Kadar et al.[53] were the first to propose combining ultrasound with hCG for accurate diagnosis of early ectopic pregnancy. They introduced the concept of the discriminatory serum hCG "zone." According to this concept, a diagnosis of ectopic pregnancy was likely whenever intrauterine pregnancy was not detected by transabdominal ultrasound at serum hCG concentrations more than the threshold of 6,500 IU/L. The clinical value of this combination was limited because many patients with ectopic pregnancy have serum hCG well under 6,500 IU/L. However, the introduction of transvaginal sonography (TVS) dramatically changed the situation. TVS can effectively detect much smaller intrauterine and ectopic pregnancies because of its superior resolution. This brought the cut-off level of serum hCG down to between 1,000 and 2,000 IU/L for those patients with sonographic findings suggestive of ectopic pregnancy. The finding of an empty uterine cavity can be associated with an ectopic pregnancy, early pregnancy, and complete or incomplete miscarriage. This should be correlated with the β-hCG level. If the beta-hCG level is less than the predetermined discriminatory level, then hCG should be measured every 48 hours and a repeat ultrasound performed when the level has reached the predetermined discriminatory level.[54] If no intrauterine pregnancy is detected when the beta-hCG is more than the predetermined threshold level or if the beta-hCG stabilizes or fails to increase normally, then the diagnosis of an ectopic pregnancy needs to be considered.[55]

Culdocentesis

Culdocentesis is performed only rarely in modern practice, because ultrasonography can reveal the presence of any free fluid in the pelvis. Culdocentesis is used primarily when ultrasonography is not readily available.[56] A culdocentesis that is positive for nonclotting bloody fluid strongly suggests the presence of a bleeding ectopic pregnancy. The finding of a yellow or straw-colored fluid is more consistent with a ruptured ovarian cyst.

Laparoscopy

The introduction of laparoscopy in the late 1960s solved the dilemma of prolonged clinical observation and the risk of performing an unnecessary laparotomy in suspected cases.[57] Laparoscopy remained the only reliable method for diagnosing and excluding ectopic pregnancy well into the 1980s, and allowed combination of diagnosis and surgical treatment.

TREATMENT

Tubal pregnancy can be treated surgically by laparotomy or laparoscopy, medically, and occasionally by observation alone. With earlier diagnosis of ectopic pregnancy has come a move toward more conservative approaches. These include surgical and nonsurgical management. Treatment must be customized to the clinical condition and future fertility requirements of the patient.

Surgical Treatment

Previously, salpingectomy by laparotomy was the gold standard for the treatment of ectopic pregnancy. A number of different approaches to conservative surgical treatment have been introduced, including excision of the affected segment, milking of the tube, or linear salpingostomy using either cautery or laser. Both radical and conservative managements may be performed by laparoscopy or laparotomy.

Laparoscopy vs. Laparotomy

The traditional treatment for ectopic pregnancy was laparotomy and salpingectomy. In the 1980s, laparoscopic approach became more widely accepted, following the development of video laparoscopy and the publication of the first series of successful use of laparoscopy for the treatment of ectopic pregnancy.[58] In general, laparoscopic surgery is the preferred approach in hemodynamically stable patients and has largely replaced the need for laparotomy because of improved postoperative recovery time and reduced morbidity.[59] Nonetheless, laparotomy is the preferred technique when the patient is hemodynamically unstable, if the surgeon has not been trained in laparoscopy, or if laparoscopic surgery equipment is not available.[60] Several randomized controlled trials (RCTs)[61–64] comparing the procedures have shown that laparoscopy is associated with shorter operation times, less intraoperative blood loss, shorter hospital stay, and lower analgesic requirements. There is no difference between these surgical approaches in subsequent reproductive outcome. However, there is a trend toward higher rates of persistent trophoblast associated with laparoscopic surgery for ectopic pregnancy.

Salpingectomy vs. Salpingostomy

At the present time, salpingectomy is used less frequently than salpingostomy. Salpingectomy is preferable in patients with uncontrolled bleeding, extensive tubal damage, or recurrent ectopic pregnancy in the same tube. It is also used when the patient wants a sterilization procedure to be performed.[65] Linear salpingostomy is the most commonly performed technique. The principle of this procedure is to open the affected portion of tube by either cautery or laser, to evacuate its content, with the incision being then left to heal by secondary intent. Salpingostomy is indicated where the patient is hemodynamically stable, wishes to conserve her fertility, there is an unruptured ectopic pregnancy of no more than 5 cm in diameter, and, especially, when the contralateral tube is absent or damaged.

Although there is no RCT comparing salpingectomy and salpingostomy, several studies have compared reproductive outcome following the treatment of ectopic pregnancy by these techniques.[49,66,67,69] Subsequent fertility, recurrent ectopic pregnancy, and intrauterine pregnancy rates are higher following salpingostomy. Persistent trophoblastic tissues are less associated with salpingectomy. The cost of salpingostomy is slightly more than salpingectomy in the short term. Additional treatment for persistent ectopic pregnancies is occasionally required after salpingostomy. However, if the subsequent need for assisted conception is taken into account, the cost of salpingostomy becomes less than that of salpingectomy.[49]

Table 6.4 Criteria for Methotrexate Treatment

A. Indications
- Hemodynamically stable patients
- Minimal or no symptoms
- Serum hCG is $\leq$ 3,000 IU/L
- No contraindications for methotrexate
- Patient are able to comply with the followup for several weeks

B. Contraindications
- Liver disease
- Renal disease
- Blood disorder
- Breastfeeding
- Presence of fetal cardiac activity
- Active peptic ulcer or colitis

C. Side effects
- Abdominal pain following treatment
- Stomatitis
- GIT upset
- Photosensitivity skin reaction
- Tubal rupture during followup

D. Dose
- Intramuscular single dose of 50 mg/m^2 or 1mg/kg in the most widely used regimen

Other Surgical Techniques

The "milking technique" is performed when an ectopic pregnancy is located at the fimbrial end of the Fallopian tube. This technique allows the trophoblastic tissue to pass through the fimbrial end of the tube. However, "milking" is associated with an unacceptable high rate of persistent trophoblast postprocedure and is not recommended.[70] When the pregnancy is located in the isthmic portion of the Fallopian tube, it is possible to excise that segment with later reanastomosis under microscopic guidance.

Medical Treatment

The effective early diagnosis of ectopic pregnancy without laparoscopy has allowed use of medical management of EP.[71] Agents used for the treatment of trophoblastic disease include methotrexate, hyperosmolar glucose, prostaglandins, and mifepristone (RU486). The most studied of these agents is methotrexate, a folic acid antagonist that is metabolized in the liver and excreted by the kidney. Methotrexate is a cytotoxic agent that inhibits the synthesis of purines and pyrimidines. It prevents synthesis of amino acids, RNA, and DNA and destroys rapidly dividing trophoblastic tissue.

Methotrexate can be administered to suitable patients by intravenous or intramuscular injection, or by local injection under the guidance of either ultrasound or laparoscope.[72] Criteria for methotrexate treatment of ectopic pregnancy are summarized in Table 6.4.[71] The most widely used regimen is to administer a single intramuscular dose of methotrexate calculated by body surface area

(50 mg/m^2) or body weight (1mg/kg). For most women this will be between 75 mg and 90 mg. Following methotrexate injection, nearly 75 percent of patients will experience abdominal pain due to tubal abortion, rise in serum hCG levels in the following 3 days, stomatitis, diarrhea, and some may need a second dose of methotrexate. Tubal rupture can still occur.[73] A serum hCG measurement is made on days 4 and 7 and a further dose is given if levels have failed to fall by more than 15 percent in 48 hours.[74] Falling hCG levels do not exclude the possibility of tubal rupture. An RCT has reported that there is no benefit of combining mifepristone and methotrexate.[75]

The variable dose regimen involves the addition of citrovorum, a reduced form of folate that blocks the effect of methotrexate, to prevent the adverse effects of methotrexate on other tissues.[76] Patients should be advised to avoid sexual intercourse during treatment, becoming pregnant for 6 months posttreatment, and excessive exposure to sunlight and alcohol. Prior to the administration of methotrexate, a clear information sheet about the adverse effects and possible need for further treatment should be given to the patient, and a written consent should be obtained.

Methotrexate vs. Salpingostomy

In general, when an ectopic sac is found at laparoscopy, either a linear salpingostomy with removal of the trophoblast or removal of the tube should be performed. In these cases, intramuscular methotrexate is indicated only when high serum hCG levels persist.[77] Several studies have compared laparoscopic salpingostomy with methotrexate injection.[73] In most cases, when appropriate inclusion criteria were used, methotrexate treatment was almost as effective as surgery with success rates of 88.2 percent and 95.9 percent, respectively. Lipscomb et al.[73] reported that 14 percent of patients treated with methotrexate required more than one dose and fewer than 10 percent required surgical intervention. The potential advantages of methotrexate are the avoidance of surgery and its complications and preservation of tubal patency and function. In addition, medical treatment may be more cost effective.

Expectant Management

When serum hCG is below the discriminatory zone and there is no intra- or extrauterine pregnancy detected by transvaginal ultrasound, the pregnancy can be described as being of unknown location.[78] Several studies have reported that 44 to 69 percent of pregnancies of unknown location resolve spontaneously. Pregnancies of unknown location may be small ectopic pregnancies, which are absorbed or resolve by tubal abortion, or early intrauterine pregnancies that miscarry. Expectant management is an option for clinically stable women with serum hCG levels below the discriminatory zone, minimal symptoms associated with either pregnancy of unknown location or ectopic pregnancy diagnosed on ultrasound.[79] Regular followup is essential. Serial serum hCG concentrations should be measured until they reach less than 20 IU/L. If symptoms and signs of ectopic pregnancy develop, serum hCG concentrations rise above discriminatory zone or start to plateau, active intervention should be considered.[79] Clear information about the importance of compliance with followup should be given to the patient if a policy of expectant management is followed.

Anti-D Immunoglobulin

It is recommended that anti-D immunoglobulin at a dose of 250 IU be given to all nonsensitized women who are rhesus negative and who have ectopic pregnancy.

COMPLICATIONS OF ECTOPIC PREGNANCY

Persistent Trophoblastic Tissue

Persistent trophoblast is usually a complication of laparoscopic or open salpingostomy, with an incidence rate of 8.1 percent and 4 percent, respectively.[80] It is detected by the failure of serum hCG concentrations to decline as expected after initial treatment. Risk factors for persistent trophoblastic tissue include high preoperative serum hCG (>3,000 IU/L), a rapid preoperative rise in serum hCG, and the presence of active tubal bleeding.[80] Currently, there is no common protocol for the early diagnosis and initiation of treatment. One study has recommended initiating second-line treatment if the serum hCG is greater than 10 percent of the preoperative level 10 days after surgery. Another study has suggested starting treatment if serum hCG concentrations are more than 65 percent of their initial levels at 48 hours after surgery. A single dose (50 mg/m^2) of methotrexate has been widely used instead of a second surgical procedure. In addition, one RCT comparing the use of prophylactic methotrexate at the time of laparoscopic salpingostomy with simple salpingostomy alone showed a reduction in the rate of persistent trophoblast by 19 percent and 14 percent, respectively.

Prospects for Subsequent Fertility

Intrauterine Pregnancy

Several studies have investigated the prognosis for subsequent intrauterine pregnancy following different lines of treatment for ectopic pregnancy. At the present time, pooled data from these studies are confusing. No RCT has been done to compare the different lines of treatment for EP. It has been reported that after expectant management, the rate of intrauterine pregnancy ranged between 50 and 78 percent.[81] When comparing conservative and radical surgery, the results are inconsistent, with intrauterine pregnancy rates varying from no significant difference to lower rates after salpingectomy.[61–64] Regardless of the type of tubal surgery, laparoscopic treatment resulted in a higher rate of intrauterine pregnancy (61% versus 53%) compared with laparotomy.[77] Despite tubal preservation, intrauterine pregnancy rates following methotrexate injection are

Table 6.5 Summary of Subsequent Fertility Following Different Lines of Treatment for EP

	Intrauterine Pregnancy	*Recurrent EP*
Laparoscopic salpingectomy	54%	8%
Laparoscopic salpingostomy	60%	18%
Laparotomy	53%	7%
Expectant management	50–68%	4.2–5%
MTX injection	54%	8%

comparable to those following laparoscopic salpingectomy (54% versus 55.5%)[73] (Table 6.5).

Recurrent Ectopic Pregnancy

Recurrent ectopic pregnancy may follow either open or laparoscopic surgery and may be secondary to adhesion formation. Several studies have compared reproductive outcome following open and laparoscopic surgery using either radical or conservative techniques. One study has shown that the rates of recurrent ectopic pregnancy were 7 percent and 14 percent following laparotomy and laparoscopy,[82] respectively. In another study, the rates were 18.3 percent and 7.7 percent in the conservative and radical groups, respectively.[66] Risk of recurrent EP is relatively low (4.2%) following expectant management.[81] While after methotrexate, the rate of recurrent EP is around 8 percent.[3]

REFERENCES

1. Hankins GD, Clark SL, Cunningham FG, Gilstrap LC. Ectopic pregnancy. In: *Operative obstetrics.* Norwalk, CT: Appleton & Lang; 1995. pp. 437–56.
2. Sau M, Sau AK, Roberts JK, Goldthorp W. Treatment of unruptured ectopic pregnancy with methotrexate: a UK experience. *Acta Obstet Gynecol Scand.* 2000;**79**:790–2.
3. Tay JI, Moore J, Walker JJ. Ectopic pregnancy. *BMJ.* 2000;**320**:916–19.
4. Department of Health. Report on confidential enquiries into maternal deaths in the United Kingdom 1988–1990. London: HMSO; 1994:61–7.
5. Department of Health. Report on confidential enquiries into maternal deaths in the United Kingdom 1991–1993. London: HMSO; 1996:68–73.
6. Simms I, Rogers PA, Nicoll A. The influence of demographic change and cumulative risk of pelvic inflammatory on the change of ectopic pregnancy. *Epidemiol Infect.* 1997;**119**:49–52.
7. Bouyer J, Coste J, Shojaei T, Pouly JL, Fernandez H, Gerbaud L, Job-Spira N. Risk factors for ectopic pregnancy: a comprehensive analysis based on a large case-control, population-based study in France. *Am J Epidemiol.* 2003;**157**:185–94.
8. Rhoton-Vlasak A. Infections and infertility. *Prim Care Update Ob Gyns.* 2000;**7**:200–6.
9. Marchbanks PA, Annegers JF, Coulam CB, Strathy JH, Kurland LT. Risk factors for ectopic pregnancy. A population based study. *JAMA.* 1988;**259**:1823–7.
10. Westrom L, Bengtsson LPH, Mardh PA. Incidence, trends, and risk factors of ectopic pregnancy in a population of women. *BMJ.* 1981;**282**:15–18.

11. Velebil P, Wingo PA, Xia Z, Wilcox LS, Peterson HB. Rate of hospitalization for gynecologic disorders among reproductive-age women in the United States. *Obstet Gynecol.* 1995;**86**:764–9.
12. Hillis SD, Owens LM, Marchbanks PA, Amsterdam LF, MacKenzie WR. Recurrent chlamydial infections increase the risks of hospitalization for ectopic pregnancy and pelvic inflammatory disease. *Am J Obstet Gynecol.* 1997;**176**:103–7.
13. Barlow RE, Cooke ID, Odukoya O, Heatley MK, Jenkins J, Narayansingh G, Ramsewak SS, Eley A. The prevalence of *Chlamydia trachomatis* in fresh tissue specimens from patients with ectopic pregnancy or tubal factor infertility as determined by PCR and in-situ hybridisation. *J Med Microbiol.* 2001;**50**:902–8.
14. Mardh PA. Influence of infection with Chlamydia trachomatis on pregnancy outcome, infant health, and lifelong sequelae in infected offspring. *Best Pract Res Clin Obstet Gynaecol.* 2002;**16**:847–64.
15. Cates W Jr, Rolfs RT Jr, Aral SO. Sexually transmitted diseases, pelvic inflammatory disease, and infertility: an epidemiologic update. *Epidemiol Rev.* 1990;**12**:199–220.
16. Hillis SD, Nakashima A, Amsterdam L, Pfister J, Vaughn M, Addiss D, Marchbanks PA, Owens LM, Davis JP. The impact of a comprehensive chlamydia prevention program in Wisconsin. *Fam Plann Perspect.* 1995 May-Jun;**27**(3):108–11.
17. Egger M, Low N, Smith GD, Lindblom B, Herrmann B. Screening for chlamydial infections and the risk of ectopic pregnancy in a county in Sweden: ecological analysis. *BMJ.* 1998;**316**:1776–80.
18. Spandorfer SD, Barnhart KT. Role of previous ectopic pregnancy in altering the presentation of suspected ectopic pregnancy. *J Reprod Med.* 2003;**48**:133–6.
19. Clausen I. Conservative versus radical surgery for tubal pregnancy. A review. *Acta Obstet Gynecol Scand.* 1996;**75**:8–12.
20. Pisarska MD, Carson SA, Buster JE. Ectopic pregnancy. *Lancet.* 1998;**351**:1115–20.
21. Peterson HB, Xia Z, Hughes JM, Wilcox LS, Tylor LR, Trussell J. The risk of ectopic pregnancy after tubal sterilization. U.S. Collaborative Review of Sterilization Working Group. *N Engl J Med.* 1997;**336**:762–7.
22. Xiong X, Buekens P, Wollast E. IUD use and the risk of ectopic pregnancy: a meta-analysis of case-control studies. *Contraception.* 1995;**52**:23–34.
23. Bouyer J, Rachou E, Germain E, Fernandez H, Coste J, Pouly JL, Job-Spira N. Risk factors for extrauterine pregnancy in women using an intrauterine device. *Fertil Steril.* 2000;**74**:899–908.
24. Franks AL, Beral V, Cates W Jr, Hogue CJ. Contraception and ectopic pregnancy risk. *Am J Obstet Gynecol.* 1990;**163**:1120–3.
25. Abu JI, Wandless GM, Emembolu JO. Ectopic pregnancy in the levonorgestrel-releasing intrauterinesystem (LNG-IUS) user: atypical presentation. *J Obstet Gynaecol.* 2002;**22**:567–8.
26. Andersson K, Odlind V, Rybo G. Levonorgestrel-releasing and copper-releasing (Nova T) IUDs during five years of use: a randomized comparative trial. *Contraception.* 1994;**49**:56–72.
27. Ojutiku D, Cutner A, Rymer J. Ectopic pregnancy with levonorgestrel releasing intrauterine system. *Br J Fam Plann.* 1998;**24**:85–6.
28. Kwong FN, Rai H, Mayne C. Ectopic pregnancy with a translocated Mirena intrauterine system. *J Fam Plann Reprod Health Care.* 2002;**28**:95–6.
29. Sivin I. Risks and benefits, advantages and disadvantages of levonorgestrel-releasing contraceptive implants. *Drug Saf.* 2003;**26**:303–35.
30. Gawronska B, Stepien A, Ziecik AJ. Effect of estradiol and progesterone on oviductal LH-receptors and LH-dependent relaxation of the porcine oviduct. *Theriogenology.* 2000;**53**:659-72.
31. Davies S, Richardson MC, Anthony FW, Mukhtar D, Cameron IT. Progesterone inhibits insulin-like growth factor binding protein-1 (IGFBP-1) production by explants of the Fallopian tube. *Mol Hum Reprod.* 2004;**10**:935-9.

30. Ferland RJ, Chadwick DA, O'Brien JA, Granai CO 3rd. An ectopic pregnancy in the upper retroperitoneum following in vitro fertilization and embryo transfer. *Obstet Gynecol.* 1991;**78**:544–6.
33. Agrawal SK, Arthur WL, Garzo G, Meldrum DR. Cornual pregnancies in patients with prior salpingectomy undergoing in vitro fertilization and embryo transfer. *Fertil Steril.*1996;**65**:659–60.
34. Ribic-Pucelj M, Tomazevic T, Vogler A, Meden-Vrtovec H. Risk factors for ectopic pregnancy after in vitro fertilization and embryo transfer. *J Assist Reprod Genet.* 1995;**12**: 594–8.
35. Strandell A, Thorburn J, Hamberger L. Risk factors for ectopic pregnancy in assisted reproduction. *Fertil Steril.* 1999;**71**:282–6.
36. Deshpande N, Mathers A, Acharya U. Broad ligament twin pregnancy following in vitro fertilization. *Hum Reprod.* 1999;**14**:852–4.
37. Azem F, Yaron Y, Botchan A, Amit A, Yovel I, David MP, Peyser MR, Lessing JB. Ectopic pregnancy after in vitro fertilization-embryo transfer (IVF-ET): the possible role of the ET technique. *J Assist Reprod Genet.* 1993;**10**:302–4.
38. Nazari A, Askari HA, Check JH, O'Shaughnessy A. Embryo transfer technique as a cause of ectopic pregnancy in in vitro fertilization. *Fertil Steril.* 1993;**60**:919–21.
39. Toki T, Obinata M, Nakayama K, Oguchi O, Fujii S. Ovarian pregnancy associated with microscopic decidualized endometriosis of the ovary: report of a case. *J Obstet Gynaecol Res.* 1998;**24**:45–8.
40. Hunter RH. Tubal ectopic pregnancy: a pathophysiological explanation involving endometriosis. *Hum Reprod.* 2002;**17**:1688–91.
41. Stergachis A, Scholes D, Daling JR, Weiss NS, Chu J. Maternal cigarette smoking and the risk of tubal pregnancy. *Am J Epidemiol.* 1991;**15**;**133**:332–7.
42. Phillips RS, Tuomala RE, Feldblum PJ, Schachter J, Rosenberg MJ, Aronson MD. The effect of cigarette smoking, *Chlamydia trachomatis* infection, and vaginal douching on ectopic pregnancy. *Obstet Gynecol.* 1992;**79**:85–90.
43. Saraiya M, Berg CJ, Kendrick JS, Strauss LT, Atrash HK, Ahn YW. Cigarette smoking as a risk factor for ectopic pregnancy. *Am J Obstet Gynecol.* 1998;**178**:493–8.
44. Milhan D. DES exposure: implications for childbearing. *Int J Childbirth Educ.* 1992;**7**: 21–8.
45. Abbott L. Ectopic pregnancy: symptoms, diagnosis and management. *Nurs Times* 2004;**100**:32-3.
46. Kaplan BC, Dart RG, Moskos M, Kuligowska E, Chun B, Adel Hamid M, Northern K, Schmidt J, Kharwadkar A. Ectopic pregnancy: prospective study with improved diagnostic accuracy. *Ann Emerg Med.* 1996;**28**:10-7.
47. Long CA, Whitworth NS, Murthy HM, Bacquet K, Cowan BD. First-trimester rapid semiquantitative assay for urine pregnanediol glucuronide predicts gestational outcome with the same diagnostic accuracy as serial human chorionic gonadotropin measurements. *Am J Obstet Gynecol.* 1994;**170**:1822–5.
48. Dumps P, Meisser A, Pons D, Morales MA, Anguenot JL, Campana A, Bischof P. Accuracy of single measurements of pregnancy-associated plasma protein-A, human chorionic gonadotropin, and progesterone in the diagnosis of early pregnancy failure. *Eur J Obstet Gynecol Reprod Biol.* 2002;**100**:174–80.
49. Mol BW, Matthijsse HC, Tinga DJ, Huynh T, Hajenius PJ, Ankum WM, Bossuyt PM, Van Der Veen F. Fertility after conservative and radical surgery for tubal pregnancy. *Hum Reprod.* 1998a;**13**:1804–9.
50. Seifer DB, Lambert-Messerlian GM, Canick JA, Frishman GN, Schneyer AL. Serum inhibin levels are lower in ectopic than intrauterine spontaneously conceived pregnancies. *Fertil Steril.* 1996;**65**:667–9.
51. Cacciatore B, Tiitinen A, Stenman UH, Ylostalo P. Normal early pregnancy: serum hCG levels and vaginal ultrasonography findings. *Br J Obstet Gynaecol.* 1990;**97**:899–903.

52. Barnhart KT, Simhan H, Kamelle SA. Diagnostic accuracy of ultrasound above and below the beta-hCG discriminatory zone. *Obstet Gynecol.* 1999;**94**:583–7.
53. Kadar N, DeVore G, Romero R. Discriminatory hCG zone: its use in the sonographic evaluation for ectopic pregnancy. *Obstet Gynecol.* 1981;**58**:156–61.
54. Ankum WM, Van Der Veen F, Hamerlynck JV, Lammes FB. Suspected ectopic pregnancy. What to do when human chorionic gonadotropin levels are below the discriminatory zone. *J Reprod Med.* 1995;**40**:525–8.
55. Bryan S. Current challenges in the assessment and management of patients with bleeding in early pregnancy. *Emerg Med.* 2003;**25**:219–22.
56. Chen PC, Sickler GK, Dubinsky TJ, Maklad N, Jacobi RL, Weaver JE. Sonographic detection of echogenic fluid and correlation with culdocentesis in the evaluation of ectopic pregnancy. *Am J Roentgenol.* 1998;**170**:1299–302.
57. Ankum WM, Hajenius PJ, Schrevel LS, Van Der Veen F. Management of suspected ectopic pregnancy. Impact of new diagnostic tools in 686 consecutive cases. *J Reprod Med.* 1996;**41**:724–8.
58. Pouly JL, Mahnes H, Mage G, Canis M, Bruhat MA. Conservative laparoscopic treatment of 321 ectopic pregnancies. *Fertil Steril.* 1986;**46**:1093–7.
59. Garry R. The laparoscopic treatment of ectopic pregnancy: the long road of acceptance. *Gynaecol Endos.* 1996;**5**:65–8.
60. Saidi SA, Simon A, Butler-Manuel S, Powell MC. Use of laparoscopic surgery for the treatment of ectopic pregnancy in the UK: a national survey. *Gynaecol Endos.* 1999;**8**: 81–4.
61. Murphy AA, Nager CW, Wujek JJ, Kettel LM, Torp VA, Chin HG. Operative laparoscopy versus laparotomy for the management of ectopic pregnancy: a prospective trial. *Fertil Steril.* 1992;**57**:1180–5.
62. Lundorff P, Thorburn J, Hahlin M, Kallfelt B, Lindblom B. Laparoscopic surgery in ectopic pregnancy. A randomized trial versus laparotomy. *Acta Obstet Gynecol Scand.* 1991;**70**:343–8.
63. Lundorff P, Thorburn J, Lindblom B. Fertility outcome after conservative surgical treatment of ectopic pregnancy evaluated in a randomized trial. *Fertil Steril.* 1992;**57**:998–1002.
64. Gray DT, Thorburn J, Lundorff P, Strandell A, Lindblom B. A cost-effectiveness study of a randomised trial of laparoscopy versus laparotomy for ectopic pregnancy. *Lancet.* 1995;6;**345**:1139–43.
65. Sowter MC, Farquhar CM. Ectopic pregnancy: an update. *Curr Opin Obstet Gynecol.* 2004;**16**:289–93.
66. Silva PD, Schaper AM, Rooney B. Reproductive outcome after 143 laparoscopic procedures for ectopic pregnancy. *Obstet Gynecol.* 1993;**81**:710–15.
67. Job-Spira N, Bouyer J, Pouly JL, Germain E, Coste J, Aublet-Cuvelier B, Fernandez H. Fertility after ectopic pregnancy: first results of a population-based cohort study in France. *Hum Reprod.* 1996;**11**:99–104.
68. Mol BW, Lijmer JG, Ankum WM, Van Der Veen F, Bossuyt PM. The accuracy of single serum progesterone measurement in the diagnosis of ectopic pregnancy: a meta-analysis. *Hum Reprod.* 1998b;**13**:3220–7.
69. Bangsgaard N, Lund CO, Ottesen B, Nilas L. Improved fertility following conservative surgical treatment of ectopic pregnancy. *BJOG.* 2003;**110**:765–70.
70. Kaczor C. Moral absolutism and ectopic pregnancy. *J Med Philos.* 2001;**26**:61–74.
71. Ander DS, Ward KR. Medical management of ectopic pregnancy – the role of methotrexate. *J Emerg Med.* 1997;**15**:177–82.
72. Jimenez-Caraballo A, Rodriguez-Donoso G. A 6-year clinical trial of methotrexate therapy in the treatment of ectopic pregnancy. *Eur J Obstet Gynecol Reprod Biol.* 1998;**79**: 167–71.
73. Lipscomb GH, Bran D, McCord ML, Portera JC, Ling FW. Analysis of three hundred fifteen ectopic pregnancies treated with single-dose methotrexate. *Am J Obstet Gynecol.* 1998;**178**:1354–8.

74. Sowter MC, Farquhar CM, Petrie KJ, Gudex G. A randomised trial comparing single-dose systemic methotrexate and laparoscopic surgery for the treatment of unruptured tubal pregnancy. *BJOG.* 2001 Feb;**108**:192–203.
75. Garbin O, de Tayrac R, de Poncheville L, Coiffic J, Lucot JP, Le Goueff F, Tardif D, Allouche C, Camus E, Chevret S, Rozenberg P, Fernandez H; GROG. Medical treatment of ectopic pregnancy: a randomized clinical trial comparing methotrexate-mifepristone and methotrexate-placebo. *J Gynecol Obstet Biol Reprod.* 2004;**33**:391–400.
76. Stovall TG, Ling FW, Gray LA, Carson SA, Buster JE. Methotrexate treatment of unruptured ectopic pregnancy: a report of 100 cases. *Obstet Gynecol.* 1991;**77**:749–53.
77. Sau AK, Auld BJ, Sau M. Current status of management of ectopic pregnancy. *Gynaecol Endos.* 1999;**8**:73–9.
78. Condous G, Lu C, Van Huffel SV, Timmerman D, Bourne T. Human chorionic gonadotrophin and progesterone levels in pregnancies of unknown location. *Int J Gynaecol Obstet.* 2004;**86**:351–7.
79. Elson J, Tailor A, Banerjee S, Salim R, Hillaby K, Jurkovic D. Expectant management of tubal ectopic pregnancy: prediction of successful outcome using decision tree analysis. *Ultrasound Obstet Gynecol.* 2004;**23**:552–6.
80. Nathorst-Boos J, Rafik Hamad R. Risk factors for persistent trophoblastic activity after surgery for ectopic pregnancy. *Acta Obstet Gynecol Scand.* 2004;**83**:471–5.
81. Rantala M and Makinen J. Tubal patency and fertility outcome after expectant management of ectopic pregnancy. *Fertil Steril.* 1997;**68**:1043-6.
82. Yao M, Tulandi T. Current status of surgical and nonsurgical management of ectopic pregnancy. *Fertil Steril.* 1997;**67**:421–33.

VII

FALLOPIAN TUBE PATENCY TESTING

Stephen R. Killick

This chapter will describe the different imaging techniques that are currently used to assess Fallopian tube patency in subfertile couples and consider their relative merits in different circumstances.

HISTORICAL NOTE

The realization that tubal patency was a prerequisite of pregnancy occurred in the seventeenth century[1,2] but clinical tests of patency, as distinct from direct observation at laparotomy, were not conceived until the twentieth century. The often-quoted Rubin test involved insufflating a gas (initially oxygen, later carbon dioxide) through the cervix. The noise of gas emanating from the fimbrial ends could be auscultated from the anterior abdominal wall. Alternatively, either shoulder tip pain or an erect X-ray was used as an indicator of gas having passed into the peritoneal cavity. By the 1950s, an ingenious apparatus was manufactured to use an effervescent tablet placed in only 4 ml of water to create insufflating pressures of up to 200 mm Hg. Manometer readings of less than 100 mm Hg were indicative of open Fallopian tubes whereas pressures of 200 mm Hg or greater were indicative of occlusion.

The development of the image intensifier in the 1960s enabled Rubin's test to be modified with the use of X-ray contrast media rather than gas. Laparoscopy and dye were popularized in the 1970s by Patrick Steptoe and others, and vaginal ultrasound was developed in the late 1980s when the first hysterosalpingo-contrast sonography (HyCoSy) examinations were performed by Ulrich Deichert.[3]

A purely physical communication has been shown to be inadequate by the universal failure of surgical procedures placing the ovary within the uterine cavity (Estes' procedure).[4] The Fallopian tube is not a mere conduit; it provides multiple essential physiological functions for the developing embryo during its passage from ovary to endometrium.

THE NEED TO TEST FOR FALLOPIAN TUBE PATENCY

Around one-fifth of all cases of infertility involve a demonstrable abnormality of Fallopian tube structure, usually a complete blockage of one or both tubes. In a similarly large proportion of subfertile couples, no definite barrier to fertility can

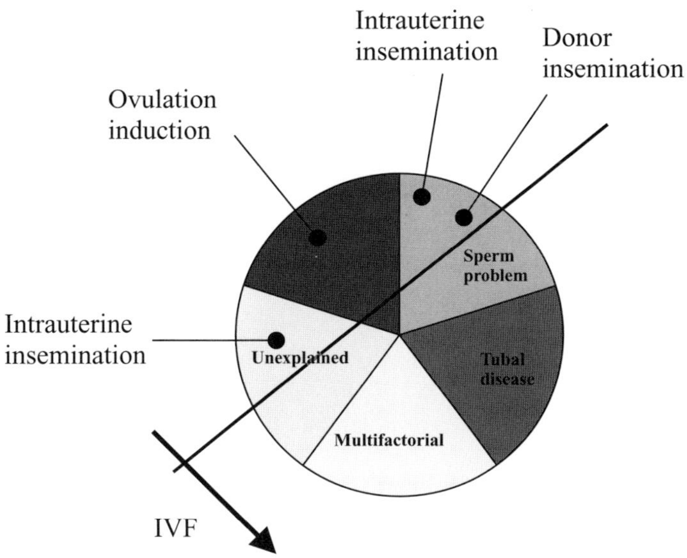

Fig. 7.1: Treatments of choice for subfertility with different etiologies. The etiology of subfertility can be divided into five groups of roughly equal prevalence. IVF provides the highest chance of pregnancy for most subfertile couples and in particular for all those with tubal disease. (See Color Plate 9.)

be identified and it seems reasonable to assume that in at least some of these cases of unexplained subfertility, abnormal Fallopian tube function contributes to the problem, even though both Fallopian tubes can be shown to be patent. We have, as yet, no test of Fallopian tube function and need to extrapolate as to whether the Fallopian tube is healthy or not from gross images of pelvic structure and demonstrations of tubal patency.

The diagnosis of a tubal factor is important because if treatment is initiated in the form of ovulation induction or intrauterine insemination in the presence of tubal disease, not only is this likely to be unsuccessful, but it also runs the risk of a tubal pregnancy. It should be remembered that infertility is commonly the result of multiple factors and that anovulation, sperm abnormalities, and tubal obstruction can all occur in the same couple. Tubal patency testing therefore should form part of a comprehensive program of investigations and counseling for all subfertile couples, unless there is a factor (such as a severe male factor requiring intracytoplasmic sperm injection, IVF/ICSI) that would necessitate in vitro fertilization (IVF) even if the Fallopian tubes were patent (Fig. 7.1). It follows, of course, that an evaluation of the ejaculate should precede any decision about whether or how to test for Fallopian tube patency.

THE TIMING OF PATENCY TESTING

As some 60 percent of women with tubal pathology have no relevant past medical history, some form of tubal patency screening should be offered to all subfertile women as soon as a semen sample has excluded a severe male factor. Hysterosalpingographies (HSGs) can be arranged prior to referral to a fertility specialist and this speeds up the investigation process.[5]

Tests of tubal patency are usually performed in the follicular phase of the cycle after menstruation has ceased. Not only might the contrast medium or

X-rays be embryo-toxic, but dye or contrast medium flowing through the Fallopian tube might flush an early embryo away from the uterus into the peritoneal cavity (although it should be said that no ectopic pregnancies have been reported to have occurred after such an event). There is also the concern that a thick secretory endometrium or menstrual tissue might impede the flow of dye through the intramural part of the tube, leading to a false-positive result. In women with an irregular cycle, ultrasound has the advantage of being able to assess endometrial development and to predict whether ovulation has occurred. In some cases, a pregnancy test is appropriate immediately prior to testing and some practitioners advocate barrier methods of contraception throughout the entire cycle if an X-ray HSG is performed.

Theoretically, embolization of oil-based media can be hazardous,[6] but this seems no more likely to occur immediately postmenstrually[7] as has been suggested.

RISK OF INFECTION

The risk of introducing infection by instilling dye or contrast medium through the cervix is low, although the procedures should be performed aseptically. Studies have shown the incidence of chlamydial infection in women attending for infertility investigations to be only 1.9 percent[8] and for only 50 percent of clinicians to use prophylactic antibiotics,[9] but these figures differ greatly from region to region. Currently published guidelines are unclear,[10] but it seems appropriate that prophylactic antibiotic therapy should be given at least for patients with a history of genital tract infection, probably in the form of a single dose of azithromycin if this is available.

PAIN

The level of pain experienced by women undergoing either X-ray HSG or HyCoSy is variable but usually minimal. Most comparative studies have shown no difference between the procedures with regard to the pain experienced,[11,12] with about 8 to 15 percent of patients experiencing significant pain enough to warrant analgesia. In our own unit, more than 1,000 consecutive HyCoSy procedures have been performed without the use of narcotic analgesics, but others have found their use necessary in as many as 19 percent of cases and even the need to resort to methods of resuscitation in 6 percent.[13] Pain can be minimized by less force of instillation, the use of lower volumes of contrast medium, warming the contrast medium,[14] early administration of oral analgesia, and confident reassurance. Intravenous antispasmodics have been advocated to reduce tubal spasm and hence aid diagnosis, but they seem to have little effect on the pain of the procedure. Blocked tubes may increase the pressure used and hence the pain, particularly if the blockage is proximal.[11] Distending the uterine cavity is painful and therefore catheters with a balloon need to be inflated slowly and carefully. Intrauterine[15] or intracervical[16] instillation of local anesthetic prior to the procedure has been shown to be ineffective.

Structural features in the female pelvis that might have an influence on fertility	HSG	Lap/hyst	HyCoSy	HSS
Patency	☺ ☺	☺ ☺ ☺	☺ ☺ ☺	☺ ☺
Endometrial polyps	☺	☺ ☺ ☺	☺ ☺ ☺	
Polycystic nature of ovaries		☺	☺ ☺ ☺	
Ovarian cysts	☺	☺ ☺	☺ ☺ ☺	
Congenital abnormalities	☺	☺ ☺ ☺	☺ ☺	
Fibroids	☺	☺ ☺	☺ ☺ ☺	
Endometriosis		☺ ☺ ☺	☺	
Peritoneal adhesions	☺	☺ ☺ ☺	☺	
Function	?	?	?	☺

Fig. 7.2: The usefulness of various imaging modalities for detecting different pelvic pathologies with a relevance for fertility. HSG = X-ray hysterosalpingography, Lap/hyst = laparoscopy and dye studies with hysteroscopy, HyCoSy = hysterosalpingo-contrast sonography, HSS = hysterosalpingo scintilography. ☺ = of some use, ☺ ☺ = quite useful, ☺ ☺ ☺ = very useful.

CHOICE OF TECHNIQUE

Fallopian tube patency can be assessed by a wide variety of imaging techniques and no one method is universally superior. There is little difference between the different techniques in their ability to demonstrate tubal patency, but they vary greatly in their ability to identify other structural abnormalities within the female pelvis (Fig. 7.2). The presence of fibroids, endometriomata, pelvic adhesions, or congenital malformations is likely to influence the treatment offered. The different techniques also differ in their cost and the expertise necessary to perform them, and some are less invasive than others.

LAPAROSCOPY AND DYE STUDIES

Laparoscopy and dye studies, or chromolaparoscopy, currently remain the gold standard for assessing tubal patency, but it is likely that this will change as improvements in other imaging techniques acquire an element of functional assessment. Although there is a need for general anesthesia, the risks are low in a young and generally healthy population. Major surgical morbidity occurs in less than 0.4 percent of cases and mortality is less than 3 in 100,000.[17] The advantages of laparoscopy include the fact that other intraperitoneal pathologies, such as endometriosis or postinfection adhesions, can be diagnosed and may explain the etiology of any tubal obstruction. Some might argue, however, that the etiology of tubal obstruction is irrelevant to the choice of treatment (invariably IVF) and that the same is true for minimal endometriosis as this is merely a variant of unexplained subfertility. Laparoscopy is obviously the investigation of choice for subfertile women with associated pain, because surgical treatment for endometriosis, should this be found, is highly effective for pain relief.

The dye used is usually 1 percent methylene blue, which is easy to visualize, very rarely the cause of allergic or adverse reactions, and appears to be safe if instilled inadvertently during very early pregnancy.[18] Methylene blue is a vital stain and hence only taken up by living cells. One study has suggested that the observation at salpingoscopy of nuclear staining of endosalpingeal cells by methylene blue could be used as an in vivo test of Fallopian tube health.[19]

CULDOSCOPY

Laparoscopy is not the only way of visualizing dye introduced through the cervix, and the current vogue is for quick, inexpensive, one-stop outpatient procedures. Inserting the endoscope via the posterior fornix (culdoscopy) is less likely to require general anesthesia but gives a more limited view and cannot be used for therapeutic procedures such as diathermy to endometriosis. Warm saline is usually used rather than the gas of laparoscopy and the knee-chest position is sometimes utilized for greater visibility.

X-RAY HSG

The use of X-ray HSG has the advantage of avoiding general anesthesia but introduces the possible hazard of ionizing radiation. A single composite two-dimensional projection is obtained, which gives excellent interobserver reliability[20] and can easily demonstrate the shape of the uterine cavity, tubal patency, and hydrosalpinx formation but little else. Good images can delineate the longitudinal mucosal folds within the ampullary part of the tube.

THERAPEUTIC TUBAL FLUSHING

The use of some kind of tubal flushing as therapeutic for fertility has often been claimed and there are even references to Rubin's test being able to improve the subsequent chances of pregnancy. This is an attractive prospect and several retrospective[21] and subsequently prospective[22] studies have attempted to show increased pregnancy rates following tubal patency testing. The most recent systematic review[23] has identified no less than eleven prospective randomized controlled trials with a total of 1,864 patients. Results suggest that the instillation of oil-based contrast material roughly triples the subsequent chances of pregnancy, but newer, water-based contrast media appear to have little effect. This would suggest that the mechanism is not simply a physical unblocking of tubal debris from the intramural part of the tube but some physico-chemical or immunological effect of the medium. The benefit is seen in cases of unexplained subfertility and in cases of minimal endometriosis,[24] implying a similar etiology in both these groups.

The most commonly used oil-based contrast medium is Lipiodol (ethiodized oil). Its precise structure is not known, but it contains ethyl esters of fatty acids of poppyseed oil and, together with all other X-ray contrast agents, huge amounts of iodine. A single HSG may result in the infusion of two thousand times the total body content of iodine.

Oil-based media are not routinely used for diagnostic HSGs because they are more viscous than the more modern water-based equivalents and cause more pain when injected because more pressure is needed. They are also more likely to extravasate during the investigation and to lead to peritoneal granulomata.

Hysterosalpingo-Contrast Sonography

The accurate and descriptive term hysterosalpingo-contrast sonography is thankfully shortened to HyCoSy.

Generally speaking, ultrasound is an excellent medium to investigate pelvic anatomy because of the multiple fluid-to-tissue interfaces around the bladder, Graafian follicle, and blood vessels. The safety, low cost, and near noninvasive nature of ultrasound enable repeated examinations to visualize structural change throughout the menstrual cycle and hence some understanding of function. The Fallopian tube, however, cannot be visualized directly.

Negative contrast media such as saline can be used to outline the uterine cavity (Fig. 7.3) and are useful to help with the diagnosis of submucous fibroids,

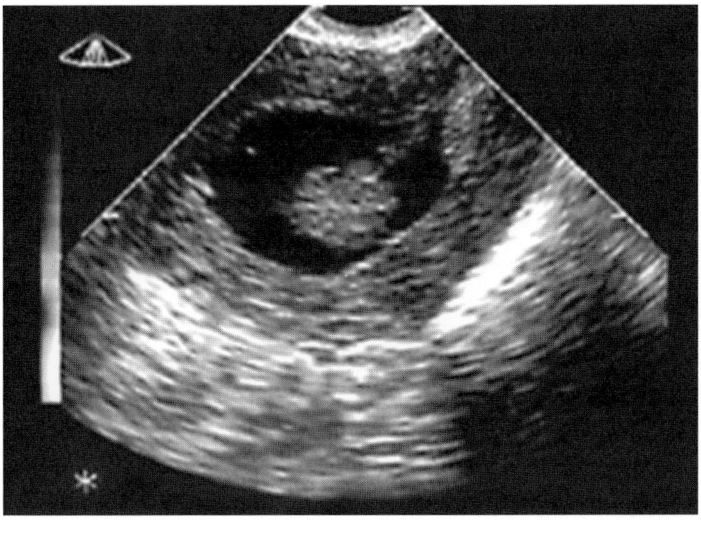

Fig. 7.3: Saline infusion sonography to reveal a fibroid polyp on a long stalk within the uterine cavity.

Table 7.1 Advantages and Disadvantages of HyCoSy

Advantages	*Disadvantages*
• Inexpensive	• Minimal endometriosis not seen
• No anesthetic	• Pelvic adhesions not seen
• No ionizing radiation	• Operator dependent
• No incision	• Learning curve ±50
• Instant result seen by patient	• False positives
• Interpretation by fertility team	
• Almost 100% sensitivity – no false negatives	

congenital uterine malformations, or endometrial polyps. Although saline can be seen to pool within the pelvis if there is at least one patent Fallopian tube, a positive contrast media such as Echovist (Schering Healthcare, UK) is necessary to visualize the tubal lumen.[25] Echovist is a supersaturated solution of galactose, prepared immediately prior to use and agitated so as to create microbubbles of air. These microbubbles are extremely echogenic and create a very bright echo even in the very narrow lumen of the Fallopian tube.

The advantages and disadvantages of the technique are summarized in Table 7.1. Particularly relevant is the direct observation of the ultrasound screen by the subfertile woman and her partner. This is an ideal opportunity to inform and to counsel. The learning curve should also be stressed, as the procedure is very dependent on the skill of the operator[26] and competency in pelvic scanning should precede any attempt to gain meaningful images at HyCoSy.[27] It has been suggested than newly trained operators should not report confidently for their first fifty procedures.[12]

HyCoSy is currently the investigation of choice for first-line investigation of tubal patency in women at low risk of tubal disease according to the National Institute for Health and Clinical Excellence in the UK (NICE[28]). If contrast medium is seen to pass through the Fallopian tubes (a negative test), the sensitivity and negative predictive value is close to 100 percent. However, if patent tubes are not visualized (a positive test), this is not necessarily due to a blockage and may be because of tubal spasm or a view obstructed by bowel gas and hence the specificity is only in the region of 75 percent. For this reason, women with a positive test result are usually offered laparoscopy with the intention of confirming tubal disease and possibly leading to a more specific diagnosis. Similarly, HyCoSy is not appropriate for confirming tubal occlusion (e.g., after attempted sterilization) when it is feared this procedure might not have been performed successfully.

HyCoSy requires expertise in vaginal scanning but it is not necessary to have a medically qualified person in attendance. Some studies have highlighted the need for analgesia or even resuscitation,[13] but our unit has performed more than one thousand such investigations in the last 10 years and no patient has required either narcotic analgesics or resuscitation (Fig. 7.4). Warming the contrast medium has been shown to reduce discomfort.[14]

One disadvantage with the HyCoSy method is that a single still image does not record the result. The uterine cavity and the left and right Fallopian tubes are

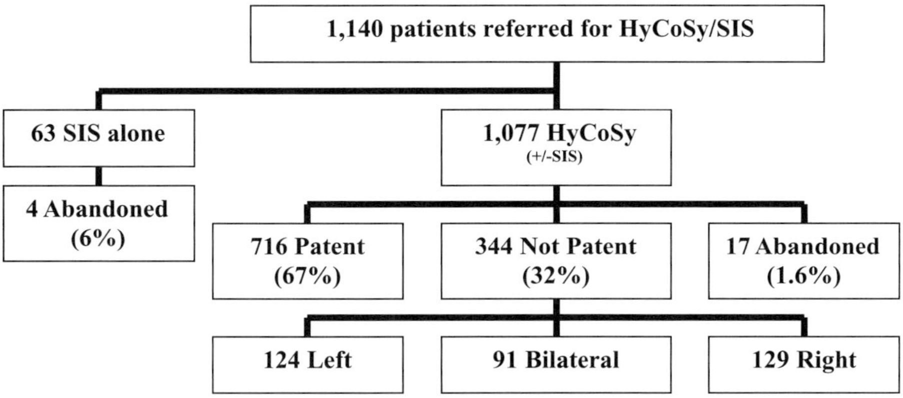

Fig. 7.4: Results of 1,140 consecutive patients referred for hysterosalpingo-contrast-sonography (HyCoSy) or saline infusion sonography (SIS) or both during the first 9 years after ultrasound techniques were introduced in preference to laparoscopy as part of the Hull Fertility Service.

never all three in the same plane and the tubes can be too tortuous to demonstrate anything but a short portion of their length at any one time (Fig. 7.5). Video recordings are necessary for a complete record although three-dimensional scanning can usually generate a useful printed image of one side or the other (Fig. 7.6). Other than for this purpose, three-dimensional imaging holds no advantage[29] for HyCoSy, but a combination of three-dimensional and power Doppler might be of benefit.

Despite this technique being promoted by national UK guidelines for all low-risk women undergoing investigation for subfertility,[28] a national survey found that only 14 percent of UK clinics used HyCoSy and 28 percent continued to offer laparoscopy and dye to low-risk groups.[30] Hence, there is a need for education and training in the technique.

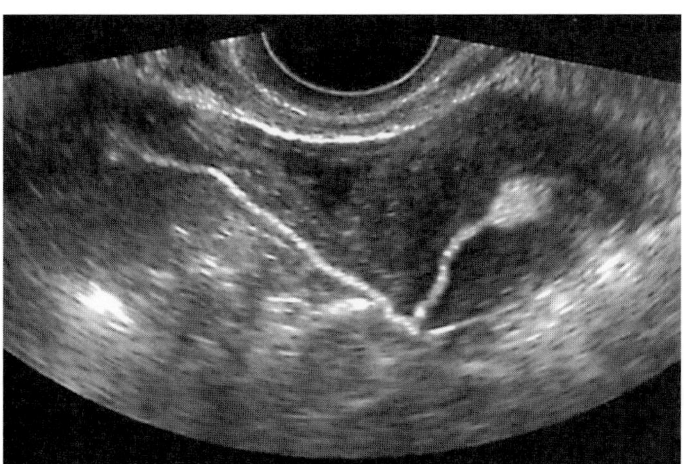

Fig. 7.5: Two-dimensional HyCoSy, which fortuitously demonstrates the entire right Fallopian tube in a single plane from uterine horn to fimbrial end.

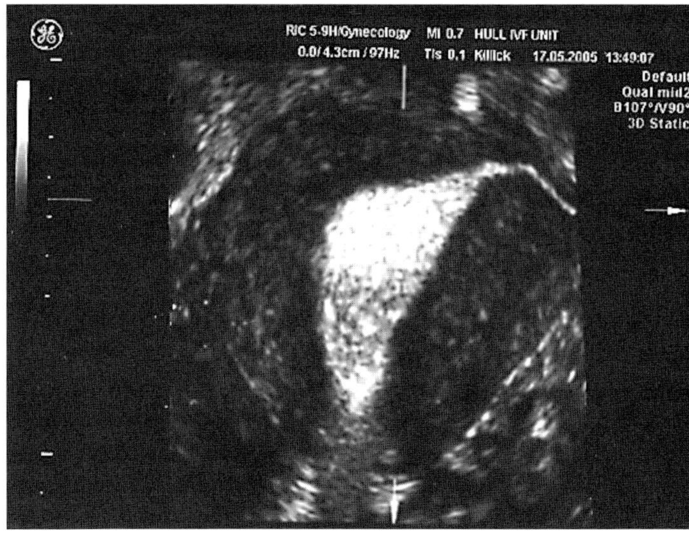

Fig. 7.6: Image generated from a three-dimensional ultrasound sweep at the time of Echovist infusion. Most of the uterine cavity and the intramural part of the left Fallopian tube can be seen, but the right Fallopian tube is in a different plane.

CONCORDANCE BETWEEN THE DIFFERENT TECHNIQUES

Concordance between either X-ray HSG or HyCoSy and laparoscopy are generally in the region of 85 percent. Taking laparoscopy as the gold standard, studies have shown HyCoSy to have a sensitivity approaching 100 percent and a specificity between 60 and 90 percent (Table 7.2). It is important to remember that the positive predictive value of a screening test is not only dependent on the specificity but also on the prevalence of the condition, in this case tubal occlusion. With a prevalence in the region of 20 percent, HyCoSy would be expected to be virtually 100 percent accurate in excluding tubal occlusion but in only about 60 percent of cases when tubal patency could not be demonstrated would the tubes be expected to be truly occluded.

Table 7.2 Table to Show the Sensitivity, Specificity, Concordance, Positive Predictive Value (PPV), and Negative Predictive Value (NPV) of HyCoSy Using Laparoscopy as the Gold Standard in Different Studies Between 1996 and 2005

	n	*Sensitivity %*	*Specificity %*	*Concordance %*	*PPV %*	*NPV %*
Chan et al. 2005[37]	21	100	67	91	89	100
Exacoustos et al. 2003[38]				86.7		
Tanawattanacharoen et al. 2000[39]	60			80		
Strandell et al. 1999[40]	43		90	80	75	88
Cimen et al. 1999[41]	18			86		
Tanawattanacharoen et al. 1998[42]	15	100	56		80	100
Reis et al. 1998[43]	44	85.2	85.2	85.2	71.9	92.9
Kleinkauf-Houcken et al. 1997[44]	126	95	85	92		
Ayida et al. 1997[45]	19			84		
Holz et al. 1997[46]	428			83.1	89.7	93.3
Schwarzler et al. 1997[47]	54	88	82	83	58	96
Dietrich et al. 1996[48]	20			82.5		

A recent audit at our unit has confirmed these figures. Thirty-six screen positive patients had a laparoscopy and dye, which corresponds to only about 10 percent of all positives. Of these thirty-six, tubal disease was confirmed in twenty-four. The positive predictive value was therefore 66.6 percent and the inter-rater in terms of individual tubal patency, Kappa = 0.54 (Moderate).[31]

CHLAMYDIAL SEROLOGY

It has been suggested that a cheaper and just as reliable test of Fallopian tube disease would be to abandon all imaging techniques and merely perform chlamydial serology on all patients.[32,33] This might miss those cases where Fallopian tube disease has resulted from infection other than chlamydia although possibly pick up early cases where the endosalpinx might be damaged but the tube still patent. It is certainly attractive from the cost point of view.

Hysterosalpingo Scintilography

Hysterosalpingo scintilography (HSS) is a technique whereby radioactive particles, usually albumen, are applied to the cervix and their progress through the uterine cavity and down the Fallopian tubes is demonstrated using a gamma camera. The images obtained are described as resembling a Mickey-Mouse silhouette, where radioactive material in the tubes resembles the ears. HSS is the only technique where no pressure whatsoever is applied to the ascending medium. Relocation depends entirely on the muscular contractions and cilial movements in the uterine cavity and tubes. It is therefore the closest thing we have to a test of tubal function, but it is only used as a research tool, not as part of routine clinical practice.

Work by Kunz et al. has shown quite elegantly that sperm transport into the tubes at midcycle is much quicker than could be achieved by sperm motility alone.[34] Radioactive albumin microspheres were seen in the Fallopian tube within 1 minute of application to the cervix, indicating an incredible speed of 2 mm per second. Time-lapse ultrasound imagery has confirmed uterine contractions at midcycle passing from cervix to fundus with a speed of approximately 2 mm per second.[35,36] The work by Kunz et al. also indicated preferential transport into the Fallopian tube adjacent to the ovary with the dominant follicle (Fig. 7.7).

FALLOPOSCOPY AND SALPINGOSCOPY

Passing endoscopes down the Fallopian tubes, either via the peritoneal (salpingoscopy) or uterine (falloposcopy) cavity, is a specialist way of assessing Fallopian tube health. The techniques are not used as a general test of tubal patency and are discussed elsewhere in this publication.

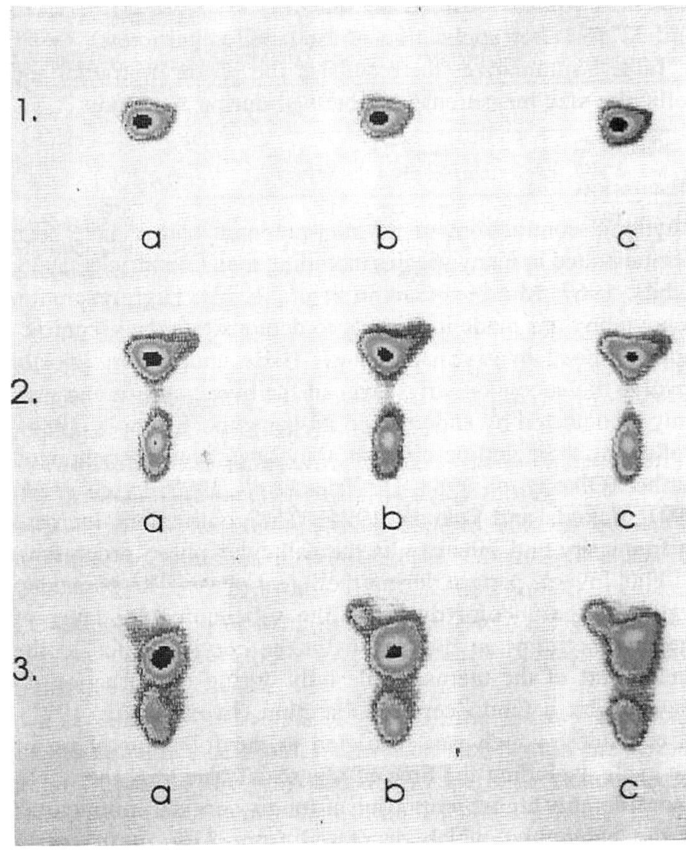

Fig. 7.7: Hysterosalpingo Scintilography in three different patients (panel 1, early follicular phase; panel 2, mid-follicular phase; panel 3, late follicular phase). In each patient, scintigrams were performed at 1 minute (a), 16 minutes (b), and 32 minutes (c) after vaginal application of radioactive labeled microspheres. With permission from Kunz et al., *Human Reproduction* 1996, **11**:627–32. (See Color Plate 10.)

CONCLUSIONS

Laparoscopy, X-ray HSG, and HyCoSy all have a role in assessing Fallopian tube patency in subfertile couples. HyCoSy is the current investigation of choice for women at low risk of tubal disease. Laparoscopy and dye should be reserved for women with additional symptoms, such as pain or women who have a high risk of tubal disease because of past history or HyCoSy-positive screening. There is a need to develop noninvasive tests of Fallopian tube function.

Note: Since the writing of this article the contrast medium Echovist has been withdrawn by the manufacturers (Bayer Healthcare, Berkshire, UK) for commercial reasons. The only remaining ultrasound positive contrast medium is Sonovue (Bracco Diagnostics, Princeton, NJ) which is not licenced for intrafallopian use but is being used for HyCoSy in some units. Sonovue contains microbubbles of sulphur hexafluoride stabilised by phospholipids and is hence both more stable and more echogenic than Echovist.

REFERENCES

1. De Graaf R. *De Mulierum Organis Generationi Inservenientibus.* Leiden, The Netherlands: Lugduni Batavorum ex officina Hackiane; 1672.

2. Ankum WM, Houtzager HL, Bleker OP. Reinier De Graaf (1641–1673) and the Fallopian tube. *Hum Reprod Update.* 1996;**2**(4):365–9.
3. Deichert U, Schleif R, Van Der Sandt M, Juhnke I. Transvaginal hysterosalpingo-contrast-sonography (HyCoSy) compared with conventional tubal diagnostics. *Hum Reprod.* 1989;**4**(4):418–24.
4. Beyth Y, Polishuk WZ. Ovarian implantation into the uterus (Estes' operation): clinical and experimental evaluation. *Fertil Steril.* 1979;**32**(6):657–60.
5. Wilkes S, Murdoch A, Rubin G, Chinn D, Wilsdon J. Investigation of infertility management in primary care with open access hysterosalpingography (HSG): a pilot study. *Hum Fertil.* 2006;**9**(1):47–51.
6. Uzun O, Findik S, Danaci M, Katar D, Erkan L. Pulmonary and cerebral embolism after hysterosalpingography with oil-soluble contrast medium. *Respirology* 2004;**9**(1): 134–6.
7. La Fianza A, Fachinetti C, Gorone MSP. Venous-lymphatic intravasation during hysterosalpingography using hydrosoluble contrast medium: a technique with no complications. *J Womens Imaging.* 2005;**7**(1):38–43.
8. Macmillan S. and Templeton A. Screening for Chlamydia trachomatis in subfertile women. *Human Reproduction,* 1999; 14/12(3009–3012), 0268-1161.
9. Glatstein IZ, Harlow BL, Hornstein MD. Practice patterns among reproductive endocrinologists: further aspects of the infertility evaluation. *Fertil Steril.* 1998;**70**(2):263–9.
10. Thomas K, Simms I. Chlamydia trachomatis in subfertile women undergoing uterine instrumentation. *Hum Reprod.* 2002;**17**(6):1431–2.
11. Korell M, Seehaus D, Strowitzki T, Hepp H. Radiological versus sonographic hysterosalpingoscopy for evaluation of tubal patency. Patient discomfort and diagnostic accuracy of HSG and HyCoSy with Echovist registered trademark 200. *Ultrschall in der Medizin.* 1997;**18**(1):3–7.
12. Dijkman AB, Mol BWJ, Van Der Veen F, Bossuyt PMM, Hogerzeil HV. Can hysterosalpingocontrast-sonography replace hysterosalpingography in the assessment of tubal subfertility? *Eur J Radiol.* 2000;**35**(1):44–8.
13. Stacey C, Bown C, Manhire A, Rose D. HyCoSy – As good as claimed? *Br J Radiol.* 2000;**73**(866):133–6.
14. Nirmal D, Griffiths AN, Jose G, Evans J. Warming Echovist contrast medium for hysterocontrastsonography and the effect on the incidence of pelvic pain. A randomized controlled study. *Hum Reprod.* 2006;**21**(4):1052–4.
15. Frishman GN, Spencer PK, Weitzen S, Plosker S, Shafi F. The use of intrauterine lidocaine to minimize pain during hysterosalpingoscopy: a randomised trial. *Obstet Gynaecol.* 2004;**103**(6):1261–6.
16. Costello MF, Horrowitz S, Steigrad S, Saif N, Bennet M, Ekangaki A. Transcervical intrauterine topical local anaesthetic at hysterosalpingography: A prospective, randomised, double-blind, placebo-controlled trial. *Fertil Steril.* 2002;**78**(5):1116–22.
17. Chapron C, Pierre F, Querleu-D, Dubuisson JB. Complications of laparoscopy in gynecology. *Gynécologie obstétrique et fertilité.* 2001;**29**(9):605–12.
18. Gerli S, Rossetti D, Unfer V, Di Renzo. Laparoscopy and methylene blue intrauterine injection immediately after undiagnosed conception: effect on pregnancy and neonatal outcome. *Eur J Obstet Gynecol Reprod Biol.* 2004;**112**(1):102–3.
19. Marconi G, Quintata R. Methylene blue dyeing of cellular nuclei during salpingoscopy, a new in-vivo method to evaluate vitality of tubal epithelium. *Hum Reprod.* 1998;**13**(2):3414–17.
20. Mol BW, Swart P, Bossuyt PM, van Beurden M, Van Der Veen F. Reproducibility of the interpretation of hysterosalpingography in the diagnosis of tubal pathology. *Hum Reprod.* 1996;**11**:1204–8.
21. Watson A, Vandekerckhove P, Lilford R, Vail A, Brosens I, Hughes E. A meta-analysis of the therapeutic role of oil-soluble contrast media at hysterosalpingography: a surprising result? *Fertil Steril.* 1994;**61**(3):470–7.

22. Nugent D, Watson AJ, Killick SR, Balen AH, Rutherford AJ. A randomized controlled trial of tubal flushing with Lipiodol for unexplained infertility. *Fertil Steril.* 2002;**77**(1); 173–5.
23. Johnson N, Vandekerckhove P, Watson A, Lilford R, Harada T, Hughes E. Tubal flushing for subfertility. Cochrane database of systematic reviews (Online), 2005 (epub) no. 2.
24. Johnson NP. A review of the use of Lipiodol flushing for unexplained infertility. *Treat Endocrinol.* 2005;**4**(4):233–43.
25. Boudghéne FP, Bazot M, Robert Y, Perrot N, Rocourt N, Antoine JM, Morris H, Leroy JL, Uzan S, Bigot JM. Assessment of Fallopian tube patency by HyCoSy: Comparison of a positive contrast agent with saline solution. *Ultrasound Obstet Gynecol.* 2001;**18**(5):525–30.
26. Papaioannou S, Bourdrez P, Varma R, Afnan M, Mol BWJ, Coomarasamy A. Tubal evaluation in the investigation of subfertility: a structured comparison of tests. *Br J Obstet Gynaecol.* 2004;**111**(12):1313–21.
27. Killick SR. Hysterosalpingo contrast sonography as a screening test for tubal patency in infertile women. *J R Soc Med.* 1999;**92**(12):628–31.
28. National Institute for Clinical Excellence, NHS. Fertility: assessment and treatment for people with fertility problems – full guideline. London: RCOG Press, 2004.
29. Watermann D, Denschlag D, Hanjalic-Beck A, Keck C, Karck U, Prömpeler H. Hysterosalpingo-contrast-sonography with 3-D-ultrasound – a pilot study. *Ultraschall in der Medizin.* 2004;**25**(5):367–72.
30. Vyjayanthi S, Kingsland CR, Dunham R, Balen AH. National survey of current practice in assessing tubal patency in the UK. *Hum Fertil.* 2004;**7**(4):267–70.
31. Landis RJ, Koch GG. The measurement of observer agreement for categorical data. *Biometrics.* 1977;**33**:159–74.
32. Akande V. Tubal pelvic damage: prediction and prognosis. *Hum Fertil.* 2002;**5**(1)(SUPPL 1):S15–S20.
33. Kodaman PH, Arici A, Seli E. Evidence-based diagnosis and management of tubal factor infertility. *Curr Opin Obstet Gynecol.* 2004;**16**(3):221–9.
34. Kunz G, Beil D, Deininger H, Wildt L, Leyendecker G. The dynamics of rapid sperm transport through the female genital track: evidence from vaginal sonography of uterine peristalsis and hysterosalpingoscintigraphy. *Hum Reprod.*1996;**11**:627–32.
35. Ijland MM, Evers JL, Hoogland HJ. Velocity of endometrial wavelike activity in spontaneous cycle. *Fertil Steril.* 1997;**68**:72–5.
36. Lesny P, Killick SR, Tetlow RL, Robinson J, Maguiness SG. Uterine junctional zone contractions during assisted reproduction cycles. *Hum Reprod Update.* 1998;**4**:440–5.
37. Chan CCW, Ng EHY, Tang OS, Chan KKL, Ho PC. Comparison of three-dimensional hysterosalpingo-contrast-sonography and diagnostic laparoscopy with chromopertubation in the assessment of tubal patency for the investigation of subfertility. *Acta Obstet Gynecol Scand.* 2005;**84**(9):909–13.
38. Exacoustos C, Zupi E, Carusotti C, Lanzi G, Marconi D, Arduini D. Hysterosalpingo-contrast sonography compared with hysterosalpingography and laparoscopic dye pertubation to evaluate tubal patency. *J Am Assoc Gynecol Laparosc.* 2003;**10930**:367–72.
39. Tanawattanacharoen S, Suwajanakorn S, Uerpairojkit B, Boonkasemsanti W, Virutamasen P. Transvaginal hysterosalpingo-contrast sonography (HyCoSy) compared with chromolaparoscopy. *J Obstet Gynaecol Res.* 2000;**26**(1):71–5.
40. Strandell A, Bourne T, Bergh C, Granberg S, Asztely M, Thorburn J. The assessment of endometrial pathology and tubal patency: a comparison between the use of ultrasonography and X-ray hysterosalpingography for the investigation of infertility patients. *Ultrasound Obstet Gynecol.* 1999;**14**(3):200–4.
41. Cimen G, Trak B, Elpek G, Simsek T, Erman O. The efficiency of hysterosalpingo-contrast-sonography (HyCoSy) in the evaluation of tubal patency. *J Obstet Gynaecol.* 1999;**19**(5):516–18.

42. Tanawattanacharoen S, Suwajanakorn S, Uerpairojkit B, Wisawasukmongchol W, Boonkasemsanti W, Virutamasen P. Transvaginal hysterosalpingo-contrast sonography (HyCoSy) compared with chromolaparoscopy: a preliminary report. *Journal of the Medical Association of Thailand.* 1998;81/7(520–6):0125-2208.
43. Reis MM, Soares SR, Cancado ML, Camargos AF. Hysterosalpingo contrast sonography (HyCoSy) with SH U 454 (Echovist registered trademark) for the assessment of tubal patency. *Hum Reprod.* 1998;**13**(11):3049–52.
44. Kleinkauf-Houcken A, Huneke B, Lindner Ch, Braendle W. Combining B-mode ultrasound with pulsed wave Doppler for the assessment of tubal patency. *Hum Reprod* 1997;**12**(11):2457–60.
45. Ayida G, Chamberlain P, Barlow D, Koninckx P, Golding S, Kennedy S. Is routine diagnostic laparoscopy for infertility still justified? A pilot study assessing the use of hysterosalpingo-contrast sonography and magnetic resonance imaging. *Hum Reprod.* 1997;**12**(7):1436–9.
46. Holz K, Becker R, Schurmann R. Ultrasound in the investigation of tubal patency. A meta-analysis of three comparative studies of Echovist registered trade mark-200 including 1007 women. *Zentralblatt fur Gynakologie* 1997;**119**(8):366–73.
47. Schwarzler P, Concin H, Wohlgenannt K. Transvaginal sonographic assessment of the uterine cavity and the Fallopian tubes with echo-enhancing agents. *Ultraschall in der Medizin.* 1997;**18**(1):8–13.
48. Dietrich M, Suren A, Hinney B, Osmers R, Kuhn W. Evaluation of tubal patency by hysterocontrast sonography (HyCoSy, Echovist registered trademark) and its correlation with laparoscopic findings. *J Clin Ultrasound.* 1996;**24**(9):523–7.

VIII

PRINCIPLES OF OPEN AND LAPAROSCOPIC SURGERY FOR TUBAL INFERTILITY

Myvanwy McIlveen and Tin-Chiu Li

INTRODUCTION

The appropriate use of surgery always depends on careful patient selection and only proceeding where clinically indicated. This will require appropriate surgical experience and careful evaluation and counseling of the patient and her partner. In the modern era of in vitro fertilization (IVF), the indications and application of surgery have become narrower. However, in expert hands excellent results are achievable in the appropriate circumstance and surgery is far from extinct. Surgery will often complement IVF treatment and thus a new era has opened up in conjunction with assisted reproductive technology.

INDICATIONS FOR SURGERY

Surgery is utilized for tubal infertility when the tube has been damaged and/or occluded. Damage and occlusion are most commonly caused by a pelvic infection or after sterilization. Tubal damage may be amenable to restorative surgery or may require IVF treatment. Surgery may also precede IVF treatment in order to maximize the likelihood of pregnancy.

STERILIZATION REVERSAL

Iatrogenic tubal sterilization should be considered separately from infectious damage. Tubal sterilization represents the group with the strongest indication for surgical treatment because of the high probability of success. Commonly, only a small portion of the isthmic tube will have been damaged, leaving the crucial fimbria undamaged. Often these women will be parous, which will also improve the likelihood of achieving pregnancy following surgery.

Up to 15 percent of women will request information on reversal within fifteen years of being sterilized.[1,2] Yet only 1 to 2 percent of patients (in North American settings) eventually undergo surgery.[1,3] Many patients will request information on reversal and then not proceed.[4] Patients are more likely to request a reversal when their sterilization was performed at a younger age and/or there has been a change in their marital status.[1,3,5,6]

In general, reversal of sterilization can be very effective if performed by an experienced surgeon, using a microsurgical technique in the appropriate patient

Table 8.1 Pregnancy Rates Following Tubal Surgery

Tubal Pathology	*Operation Performed*	*Pregnancy Rates*	*Ectopic Risk*
Sterilization	Open microsurgical reversal	50–86%	7–8%[8–10]
	Laparoscopic reversal	57–80%	3–7%[39–41]
Proximal disease	Open microsurgical reanastomosis	51–68%	10–12%[15,16]
	Selective tubal catheterization	22–47%	<5%[18–21]
Distal disease	Salpingo-ovariolysis	58–64%	2–5%[24,25]
	Salpingostomy	5–30%	15–25%[28–31,34]
Combined disease	Microsurgery	0%	12%[38]

group.[7] Younger women who have been sterilized with Filshie clips or fallope rings have excellent pregnancy rates following reversal. Pregnancy rates of up to 86 percent have been achieved.[8] This is very robust even in comparison with IVF. Pregnancy rates are lower in older women and those with coexisting fertility issues.[8,9]

Filshie clip sterilization is the most easily reversible form of tubal occlusion, because only a small area of tube will usually be damaged. Electrosurgical and Pomeroy techniques may involve damage to a considerable portion of the tube, making the reversal more technically challenging and less likely to be successful. However, pregnancy rates of 50 percent (mean followup of 8 months) have been achieved in this group.[10]

The length of tube that remains following the reversal is predictive of the chances of achieving a pregnancy and the time to achieve a pregnancy.[9,10] If 4 cm or more of tube is present, the chance of achieving an intrauterine pregnancy is better than when only a shorter length of tube remains.[9] A sterilization performed at the time of caesarean section often involves a considerable amount of tubal damage depending on the technique employed. If no fimbrial portion of the tube remains then microsurgical reversal will not be an option in any circumstance.

Older women are less likely to achieve a pregnancy after sterilization reversal.[8,9] Most pregnancies following surgery will occur within the first 12 months.[10] The possible delay in determining the success of surgery, and therefore accessing IVF, has led some gynecologists to argue that IVF should be the treatment of first choice for older women.[11] Yet pregnancy rates with IVF in women older than age 40 remain poor with live birthrates less than 10 percent/cycle started.[12] Live birthrates of 44 percent have been reported in women ages 40–45 following reversal.[13] On balance, it seems quite reasonable to offer sterilization reversal in this group of women if no other fertility factors exist and providing the option of IVF is discussed.

TUBAL DAMAGE

Tubal damage can exist for a variety of reasons. The extent and site of damage and the coexistence of adhesions will determine whether surgery is indicated.

In Western countries, chlamydial infection is the most common cause of tubal damage.[14] Previous surgery, appendicitis, endometriosis, and ectopic pregnancy can also lead to tubal damage. Salpingitis isthmica nodosa (SIN) is a histopathological diagnosis and is commonly found in resected sections of proximal tube. Its cause and natural history are discussed elsewhere in this book.

Proximal Tubal Obstruction

Ten to 25 percent cases of tubal infertility are due to *proximal tubal obstruction.*[7] Utilizing open microsurgical techniques, good pregnancy rates can be achieved provided there is no distal pathology. Cumulative intrauterine pregnancy rates of 51 to 68 percent over a 2-year period have been reported.[15,16] Approximately 10 percent of pregnancies following surgery are ectopic.[15] However, this group of patients is at risk of ectopic pregnancy even without surgery. Some studies have found lower rates of ectopic pregnancy after surgery than before.[17] Younger women and women with bilateral disease are more likely to achieve a pregnancy.[15] Surgery is often underutilized in this setting with many patients referred for IVF.

Proximal tubal obstruction can also be treated by transcervical recanalization using selective salpingography and tubal catheterization.[15] A hysteroscopic approach can also be used. It is noninvasive, diagnostic, and, in some cases, therapeutic. Its use does not preclude proceeding to open tubal microsurgery. Pregnancy rates of 22 to 47 percent have been reported.[18–21] Patency rates are higher than pregnancy rates probably due to a lack of specificity in the tool used to screen for obstruction.[22] Pregnancy rates tend to be lower when a guide-wire is used indicating the severity of obstruction if a wire is required.[19] Hysteroscopic cannulation may achieve better pregnancy rates (49%) than salpingography and tubal catheterization, but no comparative studies have been done.[23] Reported ectopic pregnancy rates have been low ($<5\%$).

Distal Tubal Disease

Distal tubal disease is responsible for the majority of cases of tubal infertility. The severity of disease can be extremely variable, ranging from minor fimbrial adhesions to complete distal obstruction with hydrosalpinx formation. Unfortunately, success rates for distal tubal surgery are less than that of proximal surgery.

In patients with fimbrial and/or ovarian adhesions, adhesiolysis can achieve pregnancy rates of 58 to 64 percent with ectopic pregnancy rates of only 2 to 5 percent.[24,25] However, this group of women does not have tubal obstruction per se but rather anatomic distortion of the tube because of adhesions. This group of patients is the most likely to be missed by a screening hysterosalpingogram.[26]

More severe distal disease with varying degrees of occlusion and fimbrial damage is less amenable to surgery. There is no universal grading system for distal tubal disease and clinicians must use their experience to determine if surgery is likely to be efficacious. In general, the degree of tubal dilation and the health of the tubal mucosa and fimbria are the most important factors in determining the likelihood of success with surgery. In patients with mild distal disease, pregnancy rates of around 40 percent may be achievable.[27]

However, pregnancy rates in patients with moderate to severe distal tubal disease are only in the order of 20 to 30 percent with up to 25 percent of these pregnancies expected to be ectopic.[28–31] Pregnancy rates are similar whether a laparoscopic or an open microsurgical approach is used.[32] Results of distal tubal surgery outside of a tertiary setting are even more disheartening with pregnancy rates of less than 5 to 10 percent.[33,34]

One of the problems with surgery for distal disease is that although patency can be achieved, this does not always restore function. The Fallopian tube is not merely a passageway but is intimately involved with early gamete interaction and embryo development. The process that has led to tubal occlusion may also have damaged the tubal mucosa. In some situations, regeneration may be possible but with severe damage this is usually uncommon. The current National Institute for Health and Clinical Excellence (NICE) guidelines recommend surgery for mild distal disease only where appropriate expertise is available.[35]

Unilateral Disease

Patients with *unilateral proximal disease* who undergo surgery have lower pregnancy rates than those with bilateral disease.[15] The assumption is that there are other underlying fertility factors as conception should be possible with a unilateral patent tube.

Up to 15 percent of patients will have unilateral distal occlusion commonly with a unilateral hydrosalpinx and a patent tube contralaterally. Surgery on the affected tube may improve spontaneous pregnancy rates by removing the toxic fluid contained in the hydrosalpinx thus allowing the patent tube and uterine environment to function normally. Unilateral salpingostomy can achieve pregnancy rates of 43 percent with an ectopic rate of 4 percent in this group of patients.[36] Unilateral salpingectomy or tubal occlusion may be even more successful with 88 percent of patients in one series conceiving.[37] The average time to conception in both series was approximately six months.[36,37]

Bipolar Disease

In patients with combined distal and proximal disease, the prognosis for surgery is poor. In one series there were no reported live births after 2 years of followup despite the surgery having being performed at a tertiary center.[38] All patients with combined disease should be referred for IVF treatment.

IVF TREATMENT

Paradoxically, one of the most common indications for tubal surgery in recent years has been to remove hydrosalpinges prior to IVF treatment. There is good evidence from randomized controlled trials that salpingectomies prior to IVF can increase pregnancy rates significantly in women with hydrosalpinges; OR = 1.75, 95% (CI 1.07 to 2.86).[42] Improvements in live birthrates are even more impressive; OR = 2.13; (CI 95% = 1.24 to 3.65). Patients with hydrosalpinges visible on ultrasound and those with bilateral disease derive the most benefit from surgery,[43] but there are improvements in pregnancy rates even in unilateral disease and less visible disease. In a Scandinavian setting, these improvements in pregnancy rates are cost effective and economics alone provide strong justification for surgery.[44]

Recently, there has been debate as to whether proximal tubal occlusion could be just as effective in some women with hydrosalpinges. Preliminary, non-comparative trials have shown pregnancy rates equivalent to those of salpingectomy.[37,45] In situations where performing a salpingectomy may be surgically challenging (e.g., dense adhesions), an occlusive approach may be easier and safer. However, this is not currently the treatment of choice because of the risk that the hydrosalpinx will cause ongoing pain and recurrent infection. Inflammatory mediators may reduce the chance of pregnancy despite isolation from the uterine cavity. In most situations, salpingectomy will remain the treatment of choice until substantive data are available validating the safety and effectiveness of proximal tubal occlusion.

In women with hydrosalpinges, careful assessment by an experienced tubal surgeon is advisable in order to decide if reconstructive surgery or salpingectomy is the best approach. There have been concerns that the widespread application of salpingectomy and IVF will ignore those patients with distal disease who may have benefited from restorative surgery. However, the two approaches are not mutually exclusive. Patients may opt for a salpingostomy initially and then proceed with IVF (+/− salpingectomy) if a pregnancy is not achieved. Indeed, the drainage of the hydrosalpinx achieved with a salpingostomy may be enough to prevent its reaccumulation and hence aid pregnancy rates through this route alone.

PREOPERATIVE ASSESSMENT

When contemplating tubal surgery for infertility, an assessment of the extent of tubal damage along with the couple's overall fertility should be made before proceeding. Prior evaluation of the anatomy and extent of disease will allow the prognosis for surgery to be discussed with the couple. Similarly, knowledge of whether there are other fertility issues will help the surgeon and couple decide if surgery is worth considering.

INVESTIGATIONS

What form of tubal assessment that needs to be made will depend on the individual's circumstances. Women who have had a tubal sterilization performed may merely require a review of the surgical technique used at the time of their previous operation. However, if there is any doubt as to the technique used or how much viable tube remains, a diagnostic laparoscopy before proceeding can be helpful. A laparoscopy will also be helpful if coexistent pelvic pathology is suspected (e.g., endometriosis).

In a patient with suspected or known tubal damage who is contemplating surgery, several imaging and investigative modalities are available to assess whether surgery will be helpful.

Imaging

Hysterosalpingography (HSG) is commonly employed as a screening tool when investigating tubal patency. It has the advantages of being inexpensive and relatively safe. The diameter of the tube can be assessed as well as the presence of rugae and SIN. HSG can also be useful as a screening tool for uterine cavity abnormalities. There is increasing evidence that an HSG will also have some therapeutic value.[46] However, it is not a reliable indicator of tubal occlusion[26] and it is of limited value in diagnosing peritubal adhesions and hydrosalpinx.[26,47] It would rarely be considered as adequate on its own in assessing whether a woman's tubal disease is amenable to surgery. Hysterosalpingo-contrast-sonography (Hy-Co-Sy) may be an alternative to HSG as a screening tool, but equivalence or superiority to HSG has not yet been determined.[48,49] Laparoscopic assessment of the pelvis should always follow an abnormal screening HSG or Hy-Co-Sy. A laparoscopy will only reveal pathology in the presence of a normal HSG in approximately 5 percent of cases.[26]

Selective salpingography, while not widely utilized, is a highly specific method of evaluating tubal patency with a low false-positive rate.[21,50] Proximal tubal obstruction is often overdiagnosed at both laparoscopy and HSG due to tubal spasm. Selective instrumentation of the proximal tube overcomes the spasm, which allows dye to pass. A see-and-treat approach can be adopted. Peritubal adhesions will be missed at selective salpingography just as with HSG.[50]

Chlamydia Screening

The use of chlamydial antibody testing has been advocated as a means of predicting tubal pathology.[51,52] The background rate of infection in the population being tested should be known in order to interpret results. Its utility in a low-risk population as a screening tool for tubal disease is uncertain.[53] Anatomical evaluation (laparoscopy) will always be required following a positive result in order to determine if tubal disease is really present. NICE guidelines currently recommend all women with infertility undergoing instrumentation of the uterus be screened for chlamydial infection.[35]

Pre-Surgery Assessment

Laparoscopy is the investigation of choice in any woman considering tubal surgery for infertility. It has several advantages over the techniques already discussed.[54] It is highly reproducible and will enable an accurate evaluation of tubal pathology and obstruction. Peritubal adhesions, combined distal and proximal obstruction, and hydrosalpinx are only reliably diagnosed with laparoscopy.[14,26] Laparoscopy can also diagnose coexistent pathology (i.e., endometriosis).[14] A hysteroscopy performed at the same time can evaluate the uterine cavity and tubal ostia. Another benefit of laparoscopy is that corrective surgery can be performed at the same operation if appropriate and with the patient's consent; a see-and-treat approach.

A laparoscopy can help to counsel the patient about the risks of more extensive surgery. Significant bowel adhesions involving the pelvic structures may make surgery more difficult and add a greater degree of risk. This in turn may alter what is planned or affect an earlier recourse to IVF.

Falloposcopy involves direct visualization of the Fallopian mucosa via a transcervical endoscope. In the hands of an experienced practitioner, it can provide an assessment of the tubal mucosa as well as tubal patency. Additionally, tubal cannulation may overcome proximal tubal obstruction in some women. Yet falloposcopy is not a commonly used tool because it has technical problems that limit its widespread use in routine clinical practice.[55,56] Fertiloscopy refers to the examining of the pelvis via transvaginal endoscopy inserted via the Pouch of Douglas. It has also not been widely adopted in clinical practice but does have some utility in the assessment of tubal damage.[56] Whether it should replace the gold standard technique of laparoscopy is questionable given the risk of bowel damage it carries.[57]

Infertility Investigations

Whenever tubal surgery is contemplated, other fertility factors need to be assessed prior to proceeding. It would be considered negligent to perform an operation with a potential for complications in a case where the prognosis was bleak or hopeless. Therefore, every couple must be thoroughly evaluated for other fertility issues before surgery is booked.

Evaluation of the female partner should include a follicle stimulation hormone (FSH) measurement on day 2–5 level. Early follicular phase FSH levels are correlated with ovarian reserve.[58] In the situation where basal FSH levels are elevated, the couple should be counseled as to the prognosis for achieving a pregnancy. Elevated early follicular phase FSH levels are associated with a reduced ovarian reserve. This in turn will have an adverse effect on the likelihood of pregnancy being achieved should tubal patency be restored. In some circumstances, the couple may choose not to proceed with surgery or may instead opt for IVF treatment. Other measures of ovarian reserve can also be utilized in predicting ovarian response. An early follicular phase antral follicle count has been shown to be a better predictor of a poor response than a basal FSH level.[59] Anti-Müllerian hormone and follicular phase Inhibin B levels are also correlated with ovarian reserve[60,61] but are currently not widely used in clinical practice.

Care must be taken in interpreting any measurement of ovarian reserve because they do not necessarily correlate well with the likelihood of pregnancy. These tests are all designed to help predict how many follicles (and therefore oocytes) remain within the resting ovarian pool. Hence, they are measures of oocyte quantity rather than quality. Although they can perform reasonably as predictors of ovarian response to FSH stimulation, none are particularly good at predicting which patient will become pregnant.

When used in the context of assessment for tubal surgery, they become even more problematic. Should a woman with a reduced ovarian reserve opt for IVF or tubal surgery? Reasonable arguments can be made for both. A patient who fails to conceive following tubal surgery and then opts for IVF has had her treatment delayed for a minimum of 6 months during which time her ovarian reserve has had the opportunity to dwindle even further. On the other hand, a patient with a diminished reserve may be a poor candidate for IVF superovulation and may be better off opting for tubal surgery where only one oocyte is necessary for ovulation every month.

A careful menstrual cycle history should help to establish the likelihood of ovulation.[14] A midluteal progesterone level should be performed to confirm ovulation.[62] If anovulation is suspected, then consideration should be given to assisted conception rather than tubal surgery. If tubal surgery is considered against the background of anovulation, it may be worthwhile trying clomiphene citrate or metformin therapy before proceeding. If the patient remains anovulatory, then surgery would not be recommended.

The age of the female partner should also be discussed in a sensitive fashion. Age is going to be one of the most (if not the most) important predictor of female fertility should tubal patency be reestablished. Age will also affect pregnancy outcomes should treatment be successful. Older women have a higher likelihood of miscarriage and chromosomal anomalies. Any older woman contemplating surgery must be realistic about her chances of success.

Any evaluation of the couple would be incomplete without a semen analysis. This should be done preferably in a tertiary level andrology laboratory competent in the assessment of sperm morphology. If an abnormal result is found, this should be repeated 2 months later to confirm the result. In the presence of a significant male factor, tubal surgery should not be recommended. Borderline abnormalities in semen parameters should be carefully discussed with the couple. If there is any doubt about the quality of the sperm, then assisted reproduction should be seriously considered.

COUNSELING AND CONSENT

In the modern surgical era, any preoperative workup must involve a thorough discussion with the patient prior to proceeding. The potential complications of surgery should be made clear and discussed in detail. The likelihood of success should also be covered in a realistic fashion. Informed consent would not be complete without the couple being made aware of the alternatives to surgery.

Surgical Complications

Laparoscopic surgery, while generally safe, has the potential for serious complications. Approximately 1 in 250 women undergoing operative laparoscopic surgery will have a complication (versus 1 in 1,000 complications with diagnostic laparoscopy).[63] In this large French series, distal tuboplasty had a complication rate of 0.35 percent or approximately 1 in 300 cases. Extensive adhesiolysis had a higher degree of risk with 1 in 100 patients experiencing complication(s). Bowel and vascular injuries are the most serious complications of laparoscopic surgery. The risk of bowel injury was 0.24 percent (1 in 400) and vascular injury 0.11 percent (1 in 1,000) in this series of operative laparoscopies.[63] The more difficult or advanced the surgery, the greater the likelihood of complications.[63] Women who have had a previous laparotomy are at greater risk of complications.[64]

Potentially less catastrophic laparoscopic surgical complications should also be touched on. Hernia formation at trocar insertion points is estimated to occur in 0.02 percent of cases.[65] The risk is proportional to the diameter of the port used.[66] Minor wound infections rarely cause serious morbidity and can usually be managed with antibiotic therapy.[66] General anesthesia is of course not without risk but is comparatively safe in this group of patients.[67] The risk of thromboembolic complications is low except in patients with preexisting risk factors.

If a laparotomy is required (or may be a possibility), then this needs to be explained and discussed. The potential for any laparoscopic procedure to require a laparotomy must be mentioned. Open tubal surgery through a mini-laparotomy will involve the usual laparotomic risks including wound infection, hernia formation, and hematoma formation. The risk of thromboembolism following benign gynecological surgery is estimated at 1 to 3 percent.[68] Unexpected bowel and vascular injury would be expected to be less likely to occur than with laparoscopic trocar insertion.

Very few direct comparisons of open and laparoscopic tubal reversal have been made. There have been no randomized controlled trials. Most of the published studies are retrospective case series and conclusions must be made cautiously. Operating time appears to be longer for the laparoscopic approach, which is balanced by a shorter postoperative hospital stay.[69]

Tubal catheterization techniques also are not without risk albeit much lower than that of laparoscopy and laparotomy. Tubal perforation occurs in around 3 to 11 percent of cases and rarely has serious consequences.[70] Hysteroscopic techniques may be associated with fluid overload syndromes if due surgical care is not taken. Uterine perforation rarely leads to adverse consequences when using a diagnostic hysteroscope.

Ectopic Pregnancy

There is an increased risk of ectopic pregnancy following tubal surgery. Five to 16 percent of pregnancies following tubal surgery will be ectopic.[8,11,24,29,31,71] The degree of risk will depend on the extent and nature of the tubal obstruction and what surgery was performed. All patients should be counseled that should they become pregnant, an early ultrasound is recommended to confirm the location of the pregnancy.

IVF: THE ALTERNATIVE TREATMENT

When contemplating surgery as a means of restoring fertility, individual patients will vary in the degree of risk they are willing to expose themselves to. IVF should be discussed as an alternative to surgery. The success and safety of IVF has improved markedly over the last 20 years. In general, success rates with IVF are going to rival or be superior to that of tubal surgery.[11] The main exceptions to this are sterilization reversal (especially in younger women), isolated proximal tubal obstruction, and minor distal tubal adhesiolysis.[8,24] There are no randomized, controlled trials comparing tubal surgery with IVF.

However, surgery does have some advantages over IVF. If tubal patency and fertility are restored this should persist beyond the first pregnancy, allowing a complete family to be achieved without multiple IVF interventions. This is particularly attractive for younger women. Importantly, there is no increase in the risk of multiple pregnancies following surgery. Many patients also find attractive the idea of surgery as a cure for their problem. Some patients will have ethical objections to IVF treatment.

Financial considerations often influence the treatment choice for patients. In many countries, tubal surgery (apart from sterilization reversal) attracts no financial cost for the patient. Yet IVF may not be free or may take years to access.

IVF and tubal surgery should not be presented as mutually exclusive options. Should one treatment fail, then the other can be attempted. Tubal surgery can complement IVF treatment. There is excellent evidence that laparoscopic removal of hydrosalpinges prior to IVF improves the chances of pregnancy.[42]

SURGICAL PRINCIPLES AND TECHNIQUE

Training and Equipment

One of the central tenets of surgery is that appropriate skill and training is required to optimize outcomes. There is clear evidence that outcomes are improved when tubal surgery is performed by experienced surgeons with specialized training.[27,34,35] The surgical skills required are often quite different from those required by general gynecologists, and it is rare to receive specialized training in the current UK curriculum. When deciding if restorative surgery is feasible, experience and training are essential. NICE guidelines recommend that distal tubal surgery in particular only be carried out where appropriate expertise is available.[35] This recommendation can equally be applied to proximal tubal surgery.

It is also important to have the appropriate surgical equipment available before proceeding.[35] Advanced laparoscopic techniques require the appropriate camera equipment and surgical instruments. Microsurgery necessitates the use of an operating microscope that may not be available in a general theater.

RECONSTRUCTIVE SURGERY

Adhesiolysis

Adhesiolysis has the potential to restore fertility and should always be considered when surgically amenable peritubal and periovarian adhesions are encountered at laparoscopy.[24,72] With laparoscopic scissors, careful dissection should be undertaken taking care to avoid damage to critical structures. Diathermy should be used sparingly when bleeding is encountered. A bloodless field is essential to discourage adhesion reformation. The principal aim should be to restore normal pelvic anatomy and allow the ovarian surface and distal tube to be freely in contact. Installation of an absorbable adhesion barrier may also be considered.[73]

Proximal Microsurgical Reanastomosis

Proximal tubal surgery has been reported as far back as 1896.[74] The advent of open microsurgical anastomoses in the 1970s as described by Winston[75] and Gomel[76] heralded a new era in tubal surgery. The use of a microscope to anastomose the tubes has several advantages. First, patency is more likely because the lumen will be more easily visualized to check its health and suture placement. Second, the finer sutures used induce less scar tissue and give a better approximation of the lumen. Third, microsurgical principles reduce the risk of postoperative adhesion formation. Pregnancy rates have reflected the superiority of this technique.

The surgical approach to proximal occlusion and reversal of sterilization is similar. The patient is placed in the lithotomy position with an indwelling bladder catheter. Broad-spectrum antibiotics are administered intravenously. A small Pfannenstiel incision is made to expose the pelvis. The pelvis is carefully packed with moist swabs to expose the isthmic portion of the tube. Careful, minimal handling of the peritoneal surfaces is important to prevent adhesion formation. Exposure and placement may also be affected through sutures placed in the round ligament and/or ovary and tied around the self-retaining retractor. Exposure is important so that when using the microscope the tubal ends sit within the same two-dimensional plane. Throughout the procedure, copious irrigation will prevent desiccation of the tissues, which increases peritoneal damage and encourages adhesion formation.

Once the surgical area is exposed, the tube is inspected and the ends to be anastomosed prepared. In the case of occlusive sterilization techniques, the Filshie clip or Fallope ring must first be removed with care. Sharp dissection with microsurgical scissors and/or microsurgical monopolar needle diathermy is combined with traction to effect the removal. The serosal surface is then incised with either scissors or diathermy at each end to be approximated.

Transection of the tubal lumen should be performed with microsurgical scissors or a scalpel (not diathermy). Care should be taken to be conservative at the initial transection. The aim should be to preserve as much normal tube as possible. Patency at the transected site should be checked with a splint threaded into the lumen. The lumen should also be carefully inspected with the microscope to confirm the presence of healthy mucosa. The proximal end can also be checked for patency with chromopertubation. If patency or healthy mucosa are not demonstrated, serial cuts of 1 to 2 mm are made until normal tubal lumen is exposed.

Hemostasis is an important component of microsurgical technique but should not be overly zealous. When transecting the lumen, care should be taken not to go into the mesosalpinx, which contains the tubal arteriovenous arcade. If these delicate vessels are interrupted, then the tubal blood supply can be disrupted interfering with healing and eventual patency. Where hemostasis is required, monopolar diathermy with a microsurgical needlepoint is usually all that is required. Microsurgical suction should be used as required but irrigation is more important.

A splint is commonly used to aid the approximation but is not crucial. This can be purpose designed or a simple monofilament nylon (Prolene) of sufficiently large diameter may be used for the purpose (1.0 or 2.0). Most surgeons remove the splint at the end of the anastomosis either through the distal tubal end or through the cervix using polypectomy forceps. Some surgeons advocate leaving the splint in place for up to 10 days postoperatively,[10] but there is no evidence that this improves patency rates.

The first suture is placed in the mesosalpinx to bring the distal and proximal ends into closer proximity. A variety of sutures have been used for this purpose. In our hands, 4.0 polydioxanone is most suitable. It is important that the operating microscope is now set up (if not already done so) in order to place the sutures in the muscularis. The microscope used must have a focal length appropriate for pelvic surgery with a comfortable stance possible for the surgeon. Magnification of X6 to X20 is usual. Magnifying lenses (loupes) are used less commonly and the choice will depend on the surgeon's preference.[77]

Sutures are then used to approximate the ends of the tube, incorporating the muscularis of both segments. Usually four sutures are placed and held until after the final suture when they are then all tied. It is usual to place the most posterior suture (6 o'clock) first but not imperative. Usually 7.0 or 8.0 PDS or nylon are used but some surgeons describe using Vicryl.[69,76]

The second layer is then closed by approximating the distal and proximal serosal surfaces. Usually three or four sutures are required. Again, PDS or Prolene are most commonly used. The contralateral reanastomosis is then performed.

Several techniques can be employed in an attempt to reduce adhesion formation postoperatively. The installation of absorbable adhesion barriers or hydrocortisone into the peritoneal cavity at the end of the operation is common. Second-look laparoscopy does not appear to be effective and increases the risks of surgery.[78] Postoperative hydrotubation with either dye or steroids or antibiotics has been tried in order to improve pregnancy rates. A systematic review showed no evidence that postoperative hydrotubation was effective.[78]

Postoperative care is similar to that of any laparotomy. Most patients are discharged from the hospital 3 days postoperatively. A follow-up HSG can be organized to assess tubal patency should the patient fail to conceive by 6 to 12 months. Patients can be advised to resume unprotected intercourse at their convenience.

Laparoscopic Reversal of Sterilization

In the last 15 years, laparoscopic reversal of sterilization has become more widely used as technology and skills have improved. Just as microsurgical techniques are not within the realm of the average gynecologist, neither will laparoscopic reversal be within the capabilities of the average laparoscopic gynecologist. Nevertheless, large series have been published with pregnancy rates of 57 to 80 percent achieved and ectopic rates of 3 to 7 percent.[39–41] One of the criticisms of the technique is the operating time required. Leaders in the field of microsurgery still believe there is a significant learning curve to be overcome before the laparoscopic technique will be adopted widely.[7]

One of the first approaches used was the single stitch technique as described by Dubuisson and Swolin[79] and modified by Bissonnette et al.[41] A four-port laparoscopy is performed with a 12-mm umbilical port and a 0-degree laparoscope. Careful dissection and hemostasis is achieved just as in the microsurgical technique. Dilute vasopressin is instilled into the mesosalpinx. The 5.0 Vicryl is used to approximate the mesosalpinx. Another 5.0 Vicryl suture is then placed at 12 o'clock incorporating the mucosa, muscularis, and serosa. Sutures are tied intracorporeally. The average operating time was 72 minutes and patients were discharged on the day of surgery.[41] Modifications involving two and three sutures have been described.[69,80] All involve incorporating the serosa and mucosa in each approximation suture.

A more traditional two-layer closure technique using a laparoscopic approach has also been described.[39] Excellent pregnancy rates were achieved (82%) with a mean time to conception of 5 months. The average operating time was 140 minutes and the authors acknowledge that the skills required are outside of the realm of the average surgeon's capabilities.[39]

Recently, a laparoscopic technique has been described that involves no sutures.[81] A 3-mm microclip is used to fixate the seromuscularis at 3 and 9 o'clock. In addition, fibrin glue is applied at the anastomosis surface. However, pregnancy rates in the initial small series published were low at 45 percent after 3 years. The average duration of the procedure was 212 minutes versus 73 minutes for the traditional microsurgical approach.[81]

Distal Tubal Surgery

Although laparoscopic surgery is not currently employed widely for proximal tubal block, the opposite is true for distal tubal surgery. Salpingostomy and fimbrioplasty lend themselves easily to a laparoscopic approach, and open surgery is rarely performed for this indication in a modern setting. There have been no comparative trials of the two approaches. Careful dissection and hemostasis are required just as in the open microsurgical techniques.

Fimbrioplasty involves removing any fibrous tissue covering the distal tubal end and freeing up the fimbria. It is the most straightforward of the procedures performed as well as the most successful.[82,83] Dissecting scissors or hydrodissection is used to carefully expose healthy fimbria. Any adhesions tethering the tube to pelvic structures should also be incised. Diathermy should be avoided unless significant bleeding is encountered. Copious irrigation is important. The aim should be to restore normal anatomy if possible.

Salpingostomy literally means to open the distal tube. However, the usual procedure is to perform a cuff salpingostomy where the distal end is not only opened but also everted in order to expose the tubal mucosa to the peritoneal cavity. The terms are often used interchangeably. This is the procedure most commonly performed when there is a hydrosalpinx.

Careful inspection of the distal tube will often enable the previous opening to be discerned. Generally, the most avascular area indicates where the tubal opening once was. If this is not the case, then the incision needs to be placed so that the opening is close to and facing the ovary to restore normal anatomy. A stellate or cruciate incision is made to open the tube. This incision can be made with scissors, diathermy, or laser. Our usual practice would be to make the initial incision with a needle point monopolar diathermy and then widen the opening with scissors. Once normal fimbriae are exposed, care should be taken not to handle or damage them. Patency should be confirmed by chromopertubation. The cuff can be maintained by suturing the newly created edge to the adjacent serosal surface of the tube. Alternatively, laser or monopolar diathermy can be applied to the serosal surface underneath the cuff circumferentially (the so-called "flowering" technique). Copious irrigation and meticulous hemostasis are important to prevent postoperative adhesions. Installation of adhesion barriers may be considered.

Unfortunately, even in the most experienced hands pregnancy rates following distal tubal surgery may be disappointing. Careful patient selection pre- and intraoperatively is important to optimize results. Patients with thin-walled hydrosalpinx and healthy mucosa have the best prognosis.[84] Tubes with gross dilatation (>3cm), thickened walls, and mucosal adhesions are generally not amenable to reconstructive surgery and IVF treatment should be considered instead.[85] Unilateral salpingostomies have higher pregnancy rates than bilateral probably by draining the hydrosalpinx as discussed earlier.[36]

Combined distal and proximal disease (i.e., bipolar disease) should not be considered for operative repair.[38]

Salpingectomy and Occlusive Techniques

In women with distal tubal disease, IVF has become the mainstay of treatment.[86] Isolating the hydrosalpinx from the intrauterine environment prior to treatment has become accepted practice.[35,42] Salpingectomy is the treatment of choice where surgically feasible. Again, the laparoscopic approach is the one most commonly taken. Occlusion should be reserved for patients where severe pelvic adhesions preclude a safe salpingectomy being performed.

Adhesiolysis may initially need to be performed to mobilize the tube. Bipolar diathermy and incision along the mesosalpinx will effect safe removal of the affected tube. Alternatively, endo-loops can be used to lasso the hydrosalpinx. The tube is most easily removed in an endo-pouch through the suprapubic port. It can also be brought out through the umbilical port without the use of a pouch. Copious irrigation and careful hemostasis are important.

Several techniques can be used to occlude the proximal tubal end. Application of a Filshie clip is the simplest. Bipolar diathermy and cut is also relatively straightforward. With both techniques, care should be taken that the occlusion is effected above the proximal end of the hydrosalpinx as close to the uterus as possible.

Transvaginal aspiration of the hydrosalpinx is not recommended. It risks introducing infection and has not been shown to be effective.[87] Reaccumulation of fluid can occur in as little as 2 days.[88]

Tubal Cannulation Techniques

These innovative techniques can be used both diagnostically and therapeutically for suspected proximal tubal obstruction. Their use does not preclude open surgery if proximal obstruction is confirmed that is unable to be recanalized.

Selective salpingography is when a catheter is passed through the proximal tubal ostium and contrast is injected locally under fluoroscopic guidance. Higher local pressures may overcome tubal spasm and mucus plugging. This technique can be performed as an outpatient or in combination with laparoscopy. Several catheter systems are available, such as the Novy cornual cannulation set (Cook Medical, Australia).

Hysteroscopic tubal cannulation is similar to the previously discussed techniques. A catheter is introduced into the tubal ostia under direct vision. The catheter is threaded through the operating channel of the hysteroscope. Patency is confirmed either fluoroscopically or under laparoscopic direct vision.

SUMMARY

Tubal surgery remains a useful weapon in the reproductive surgeon's armamentarium that should not be automatically overlooked in favor of IVF. In experienced hands and for the right indications, pregnancy rates are very competitive with IVF. Surgery can be used to complement IVF treatment and the two approaches are not mutually exclusive. Careful patient counseling prior to surgery allows the patient to make an informed decision about her options. Modern techniques such as laparoscopic reanastomosis and selective salpingography are ushering in a new era of tubal surgery. As with all surgical ventures, experience, appropriate patient selection, suitable equipment, and meticulous technique are paramount in maximizing an optimal outcome.

REFERENCES

1. Schmidt JE, Hillis SD, Marchbanks PA, Jeng G, Peterson HB. Requesting information about and obtaining reversal after tubal sterilization: findings from the U.S. Collaborative Review of Sterilization. *Fertil Steril.* 2000;**74**(5):892–8.
2. Jamieson DJ, Kaufman SC, Costello C, et al. A comparison of women's regret after vasectomy versus tubal sterilization. *Obstet Gynecol.* 2002;**99**(6):1073–9.
3. Trussell J, Guilbert E, Hedley A. Sterilization failure, sterilization reversal, and pregnancy after sterilization reversal in Quebec. *Obstet Gynecol.* 2003;**101**(4):677–84.
4. Brooks J, Taylor PJ, Freedman B, Pattinson HA. The fate of women requesting reversal of tubal sterilization. *Fertil Steril.* 1987;**47**(5):876–8.
5. Winston RM. Why 103 women asked for reversal of sterilisation. *Br Med J.* 1977;**2**(6082):305–7.
6. Platz-Christensen JJ, Tronstad SE, Johansson O, Carlsson SA. Evaluation of regret after tubal sterilization. *BJOG.* 1992;**38**(3):223–6.

7. Sacks G, Trew G. Reconstruction, destruction, and IVF: dilemmas in the art of tubal surgery. *BJOG.* 2004;**111**(11):1174–81.
8. Hanafi MM. Factors affecting the pregnancy rate after microsurgical reversal of tubal ligation. *Fertil Steril.* 2003;**80**(2):434–40.
9. Rouzi AA, Mackinnon M, McComb PF. Predictors of success of reversal of sterilization. *Fertil Steril.* 1995;**64**(1):29–36.
10. Kim SH, Shin CJ, Kim JG, Moon SY, Lee JY, Chang YS. Microsurgical reversal of tubal sterilization: a report on 1,118 cases. *Fertil Steril.* 1997;**68**(5):865–70.
11. Benadiva CA, Kligman I, Davis O, Rosenwaks Z. In vitro fertilization versus tubal surgery: is pelvic reconstructive surgery obsolete? *Fertil Steril.* 1995;**64**(6):1051–61.
12. Human Fertilisation and Embryology Authority (HFEA). National IVF Summary Statistics. 2005.
13. Trimbos-Kemper TC. Reversal of sterilization in women over 40 years of age: a multicenter survey in The Netherlands. *Fertil Steril.* 1990;**53**(3):575–7.
14. Speroff L, Fritz M. *Clinical gynecologic endocrinology and infertility.* 7th ed. Philadelphia: Lippincott Williams and Wilkins, 2005.
15. Dubuisson JB, Chapron C, Ansquer Y, Vacher-Lavenu MC. Proximal tubal occlusion: is there an alternative to microsurgery? *Hum Reprod.* 1997;**12**(4):692–8.
16. Gillett WR, Clarke RH, Herbison GP. First and subsequent pregnancies after tubal microsurgery: evaluation of the fertility index. *Fertil Steril.*1997;**68**(6):1033–42.
17. Awartani K, McComb PF. Microsurgical resection of nonocclusive salpingitis isthmica nodosa is beneficial. *Fertil Steril.* 2003;**79**(5):1199–1203.
18. Confino E, Tur-Kaspa I, DeCherney A, et al. Transcervical balloon tuboplasty. A multicenter study. *JAMA.* 1990;**264**(16):2079–82.
19. Woolcott R, Petchpud A, O'Donnell P, Stanger J. Differential impact on pregnancy rate of selective salpingography, tubal catheterization, and wire-guide recanalization in the treatment of proximal fallopian tube obstruction. *Hum Reprod.* 1995;**10**(6):1423–6.
20. Thurmond AS, Rosch J. Nonsurgical fallopian tube recanalization for treatment of infertility. *Radiology.* 1990;**174**(2):371–4.
21. Papaioannou S, Afnan M, Girling AJ, et al. Diagnostic and therapeutic value of selective salpingography and tubal catheterization in an unselected infertile population. *Fertil Steril.* 2003;**79**(3):613–17.
22. Al-Jaroudi D, Herba MJ, Tulandi T. Reproductive performance after selective tubal catheterization. *J Minim Invasive Gynecol.* 2005;**12**(2):150–2.
23. Honore GM, Holden AEC, Schenken RS. Pathophysiology and management of proximal tubal blockage. *Fertil Steril.* 1999;**71**(5):785–95.
24. Gomel V. Salpingo-ovariolysis by laparoscopy in infertility. *Fertil Steril.* 1983;**40**(5):607–11.
25. Donnez J, Casanas-Roux F. Prognostic factors of fimbrial microsurgery. *Fertil Steril.* 1986;**46**(2):200–4.
26. Swart P, Mol BW, Van Der Veen F, van Beurden M, Redekop WK, Bossuyt PM. The accuracy of hysterosalpingography in the diagnosis of tubal pathology: a meta-analysis. *Fertil Steril.* 1995;**64**(3):486–91.
27. Singhal V, Li TC, Cooke ID. An analysis of factors influencing the outcome of 232 consecutive tubal microsurgery cases. *Br J Obstet Gynaecol.* 1991;**98**(7):628–36.
28. Winston RM, Margara RA. Microsurgical salpingostomy is not an obsolete procedure. *BJOG.* 1991;**98**(7):637–42.
29. Dlugi AM, Reddy S, Saleh WA, Mersol-Barg MS, Jacobsen G. Pregnancy rates after operative endoscopic treatment of total (neosalpingostomy) or near total (salpingostomy) distal tubal occlusion. *Fertil Steril.* 1994;**62**(5):913–20.
30. Canis M, Mage G, Pouly JL, Manhes H, Wattiez A, Bruhat MA. Laparoscopic distal tuboplasty: report of 87 cases and a 4-year experience. *Fertil Steril.* 1991;**56**(4):616–21.
31. Taylor RC, Berkowitz J, McComb PF. Role of laparoscopic salpingostomy in the treatment of hydrosalpinx. *Fertil Steril.* 2001;**75**(3):594–600.

32. Dubuisson JB, Bouquet de Joliniere J, Aubriot FX, Darai E, Foulot H, Mandelbrot L. Terminal tuboplasties by laparoscopy: 65 consecutive cases. *Fertil Steril.* 1990;**54**(3): 401–3.
33. Dunphy BC, Woodhead S, Platt H, Pattinson HA, Greene C, Camenzind A. Outcome study using an administrative database: terminal salpingostomy, physician caseload, and live birthrates. *Hum Reprod.* 1996;**11**(1):77–80.
34. Watson AJ, Gupta JK, O'Donovan P, Dalton ME, Lilford RJ. The results of tubal surgery in the treatment of infertility in two nonspecialist hospitals. *BJOG.* 1990;**97**(7):561–8.
35. National Institute for Health and Clinical Excellence. Fertility: assessment and treatment for people with fertility problems. 2004.
36. McComb PF, Taylor RC. Pregnancy outcome after unilateral salpingostomy with a contralateral patent oviduct. *Fertil Steril.* 2001;**76**(6):1278–9.
37. Sagoskin AW, Lessey BA, Mottla GL, et al. Salpingectomy or proximal tubal occlusion of unilateral hydrosalpinx increases the potential for spontaneous pregnancy. *Hum Reprod.* 2003;**18**(12):2634–7.
38. Patton PE, Williams TJ, Coulam CB. Results of microsurgical reconstruction in patients with combined proximal and distal tubal occlusion: double obstruction. *Fertil Steril.* 1987;**48**(4):670–4.
39. Yoon TK, Sung HR, Kang HG, Cha SH, Lee CN, Cha KY. Laparoscopic tubal anastomosis: fertility outcome in 202 cases. *Fertil Steril.* 1999;**72**(6):1121–6.
40. Ribeiro SC, Tormena RA, Giribela CG, Izzo CR, Santos NC, Pinotti JA. Laparoscopic tubal anastomosis. *Int J Gynecol Obstet.* 2004;**84**(2):142–6.
41. Bissonnette F, Lapensee L, Bouzayen R. Outpatient laparoscopic tubal anastomosis and subsequent fertility. *Fertil Steril.* 1999;**72**(3):549–52.
42. Johnson NP, Mak W, Sowter MC. Surgical treatment for tubal disease in women due to undergo in vitro fertilisation. [update of Cochrane Database Syst Rev. 2001;(3):CD002125; PMID: 11687014]. *Cochrane Database of Systematic Reviews.* 2004;**3**.
43. Strandell A, Lindhard A, Waldenstrom U, Thorburn J, Janson PO, Hamberger L. Hydrosalpinx and IVF outcome: a prospective, randomized multicentre trial in Scandinavia on salpingectomy prior to IVF. *Hum Reprod.* 1999;**14**(11):2762–9.
44. Strandell A, Lindhard A, Eckerlund I. Cost–effectiveness analysis of salpingectomy prior to IVF, based on a randomized controlled trial. *Hum Reprod.* 2005;**20**:3284–92.
45. Surrey ES, Schoolcraft WB. Laparoscopic management of hydrosalpinges before in vitro fertilization-embryo transfer: salpingectomy versus proximal tubal occlusion. *Fertil Steril.* 2001;**75**(3):612–17.
46. Johnson N, Vandekerckhove P, Watson A, Lilford R, Harada T, Hughes E. Tubal flushing for subfertility. *Cochrane Database of Systematic Reviews.* 2005;**2**.
47. Mol BW, Swart P, Bossuyt PM, van Beurden M, Van Der Veen F. Reproducibility of the interpretation of hysterosalpingography in the diagnosis of tubal pathology. *Hum Reprod.* 1996;**11**(6):1204–8.
48. Dijkman AB, Mol BW, Van Der Veen F, Bossuyt PM, Hogerzeil HV. Can hysterosalpingo-contrast-sonography replace hysterosalpingography in the assessment of tubal subfertility? *Eur J Radiol.* 2000;**35**(1):44–8.
49. Ayida G, Kennedy S, Barlow D, Chamberlain P. A comparison of patient tolerance of hysterosalpingo-contrast sonography (HyCoSy) with Echovist-200 and X-ray hysterosalpingography for outpatient investigation of infertile women. *Ultrasound Obstet Gynecol.* 1996;**7**(3):201–4.
50. Woolcott R, Fisher S, Thomas J, Kable W. A randomized, prospective, controlled study of laparoscopic dye studies and selective salpingography as diagnostic tests of Fallopian tube patency. *Fertil Steril.* 1999;**72**(5):879–84.
51. Land JA, Evers JL, Goossens VJ. How to use Chlamydia antibody testing in subfertility patients. *Hum Reprod.* 1998;**13**(4):1094–8.

52. Mol BW, Dijkman B, Wertheim P, Lijmer J, Van Der Veen F, Bossuyt PM. The accuracy of serum chlamydial antibodies in the diagnosis of tubal pathology: a meta-analysis. *Fertil Steril.* 1997;**67**(6):1031–7.
53. Johnson NP, Taylor K, Nadgir AA, Chinn DJ, Taylor PJ. Can diagnostic laparoscopy be avoided in routine investigation for infertility? *BJOG.* 2000;**107**(2):174–8.
54. Opsahl MS, Miller B, Klein TA. The predictive value of hysterosalpingography for tubal and peritoneal infertility factors. *Fertil Steril.* 1993;**60**(3):444–8.
55. Lundberg S, Rasmussen C, Berg AA, Lindblom B. Falloposcopy in conjunction with laparoscopy: possibilities and limitations. *Hum Reprod.* 1998;**13**(6):1490–2.
56. Rimbach S, Bastert G, Wallwiener D. Technical results of falloposcopy for infertility diagnosis in a large multicentre study. *Hum Reprod.* 2001;**16**(5):925–30.
57. Gordts S, Watrelot A, Campo R, Brosens I. Risk and outcome of bowel injury during transvaginal pelvic endoscopy. *Fertil Steril.* 1238;**76**(6):1238–41.
58. Toner JP, Philput CB, Jones GS, Muasher SJ. Basal follicle-stimulating hormone level is a better predictor of in vitro fertilization performance than age. *Fertil Steril.* 1991;**55**(4):784–91.
59. Hendriks DJ, Mol BW, Bancsi LF, Te Velde ER, Broekmans FJ. Antral follicle count in the prediction of poor ovarian response and pregnancy after in vitro fertilization: a meta-analysis and comparison with basal follicle-stimulating hormone level. *Fertil Steril.* 2005;**83**(2):291–301.
60. Fanchin R, Schonauer LM, Righini C, Guibourdenche J, Frydman R, Taieb J. Serum anti-Müllerian hormone is more strongly related to ovarian follicular status than serum inhibin B, estradiol, FSH, and LH on day 3. *Hum Reprod.* 2003;**18**(2):323–7.
61. Seifer DB, Lambert-Messerlian G, Hogan JW, Gardiner AC, Blazar AS, Berk CA. Day 3 serum inhibin-B is predictive of assisted reproductive technologies outcome. [*see comment*]. *Fertil Steril.* 1997;**67**(1):110–14.
62. Wathen NC, Perry L, Lilford RJ, Chard T. Interpretation of single progesterone measurement in diagnosis of anovulation and defective luteal phase: observations on analysis of the normal range. *Br Med J Clin Res Ed.* 1984;**288**(6410):7–9.
63. Chapron C, Querleu D, Bruhat MA, et al. Surgical complications of diagnostic and operative gynaecological laparoscopy: a series of 29,966 cases. *Hum Reprod.* 1998;**13**(4):867–72.
64. Rafii A, Camatte S, Lelievre L, Darai E, Lecuru F. Previous abdominal surgery and closed entry for gynaecological laparoscopy: a prospective study. *BJOG.* 2005;**112**(1): 100–2.
65. Montz FJ, Holschneider CH, Munro MG. Incisional hernia following laparoscopy: a survey of the American Association of Gynecologic Laparoscopists. *Obstet Gynecol.* 1994;**84**(5):881–4.
66. Munro MG. Laparoscopic access: complications, technologies, and techniques. *Curr Opin Obstet Gynecol.* 2002;**14**(4):365–74.
67. Jenkins K, Baker AB. Consent and anaesthetic risk. [*see comment*]. *Anaesthesia.* 2003;**58**(10):962–84.
68. Madden SM, Porter TF. Deep venous thrombosis: prophylaxis in gynecology. *Clin Obstet Gynecol. December* 1999;**42**(4):895.
69. Cha SH, Lee MH, Kim JH, Lee CN, Yoon TK, Cha KY. Fertility outcome after tubal anastomosis by laparoscopy and laparotomy. *J Am Assoc Gynecol Laparosc.* 2001;**8**(3):348–52.
70. Martensson O, Nilsson B, Ekelund L, Johansson J, Wickman G. Selective salpingography and fluoroscopic transcervical salpingoplasty for diagnosis and treatment of proximal fallopian tube occlusions. *Acta Obstet Gynecol Scand.* 1993;**72**(6):458–64.
71. Lavy G, Diamond MP, DeCherney AH. Pregnancy following tubocornual anastomosis. *Fertil Steril.* 1986;**46**(1):21–5.
72. Tulandi T, Collins JA, Burrows E, et al. Treatment-dependent and treatment-independent pregnancy among women with periadnexal adhesions. [erratum appears

in *Am J Obstet Gynecol.* 1990 Jul;**163**(1 Pt 1):271]. *Am J Obstet Gynecol.* 1990;162(2): 354–7.

73. diZerega GS, Verco SJ, Young P, et al. A randomized, controlled pilot study of the safety and efficacy of 4% icodextrin solution in the reduction of adhesions following laparoscopic gynaecological surgery. *Hum Reprod.* 2002;**17**(4):1031–8.
74. Siegler AM, Hellman LM. Tubal plastic surgery; report of a survey. *Fertil Steril.* 1956;**7**(2):170–7.
75. Winston RM. Microsurgical tubocornual anastomosis for reversal of sterilisation. *Lancet.* 1977;**1**(8006):284–5.
76. Gomel V. Tubal reanastomosis by microsurgery. *Fertil Steril.* 1977;**28**(1):59–65.
77. Watson A, Vandekerckhove P, Lilford R. Techniques for pelvic surgery in subfertility. *Cochrane Database Syst Rev.* 2000(2):CD000221.
78. Johnson NP, Watson A. Postoperative procedures for improving fertility following pelvic reproductive surgery. *Cochrane Database Syst Rev.* 2000(2):CD001897.
79. Dubuisson JB, Swolin K. Laparoscopic tubal anastomosis (the one stitch technique): preliminary results. *Hum Reprod.* 1995;**10**(8):2044–6.
80. Reich H, McGlynn F, Parente C, Sekel L, Levie M. Laparoscopic tubal anastomosis. *J Am Assoc Gynecol Laparosc.* 1993;**1**(1):16–19.
81. Wiegerinck MAHM, Roukema M, van Kessel PH, Mol BWJ. Sutureless re-anastomosis by laparoscopy versus microsurgical re-anastomosis by laparotomy for sterilization reversal: a matched cohort study. *Hum Reprod.* 2005;**20**(8):2355–8.
82. Gomel V, Wang I. Laparoscopic surgery for infertility therapy. *Curr Opin Obstet Gynecol.* 1994;**6**(2):141–8.
83. Audebert AJ, Pouly JL, Von Theobald P. Laparoscopic fimbrioplasty: an evaluation of 35 cases. *Hum Reprod.* 1998;**13**(6):1496–9.
84. Vasquez G, Boeckx W, Brosens I. No correlation between peritubal and mucosal adhesions in hydrosalpinges. *Fertil Steril.* 1995;**64**(5):1032–3.
85. Hull MG, Fleming CF. Tubal surgery versus assisted reproduction: assessing their role in infertility therapy. *Curr Opin Obstet Gynecol.* 1995;**7**(3):160–7.
86. Aboulghar MA, Mansour RT, Serour GI. Controversies in the modern management of hydrosalpinx. *Hum Reprod Update.* 1998;**4**(6):882–90.
87. Aboulghar MA, Mansour RT, Serour GI, Sattar MA, Awad MM, Amin Y. Transvaginal ultrasonic needle guided aspiration of pelvic inflammatory cystic masses before ovulation induction for in vitro fertilization. *Fertil Steril.* 1990;**53**(2):311–14.
88. Bloechle M, Schreiner T, Lisse K. Recurrence of hydrosalpinges after transvaginal aspiration of tubal fluid in an IVF cycle with development of a serometra. *Hum Reprod.* 1997;**12**(4):703–5.

IX

IVF AND TUBAL DISEASE

Chun Y. Ng and Geoffrey H. Trew

IVF AND TUBAL DISEASE

Patent and functional Fallopian tubes are necessary for normal human conception to occur. The Fallopian tubes are highly specialized and serve a number of essential functions in the reproductive process. First, they are responsible for the critical role of picking up an ovum when it is discharged from the rupturing ovarian follicle and transferring the ovum into the tubal lumen. Second, the Fallopian tube provides an environment for sperm capacitation and ovum fertilization to occur, and finally it transfers the fertilized cleaving embryo into the uterus after an interval of 3 to 4 days.[1] Unidirectional beating of the tubal cilia and peristaltic contractions of the tubal muscles create a current within the tubal lumen to transport the ovum and subsequently the embryo. The secretory elements of the tubal mucosa are modified during a normal menstrual cycle. The production of fluid in the Fallopian tube is greatest immediately before ovulation.[2] Secretions from the tubal epithelium facilitate fertilization and nourish the embryo.[3]

Tubal and/or adhesions factor account for 25 to 35 percent of infertility cases.[4] Tubal infertility is associated with sexually transmitted diseases, multiple sexual partners, early age at first intercourse, race, socioeconomic and marital status, level of education, previous use of contraceptive methods, septic abortion, smoking, alcoholism, and abdominal or pelvic surgery.[5] Tubal factor infertility may be transient or permanent and may involve the proximal, distal, or entire tube.[6] The Fallopian tubes are very vulnerable to infection and surgical damage, which may impair function by affecting the delicate fimbriae or the highly specialized inner micro-architecture.

CAUSES OF TUBAL DISEASE THAT AFFECT FERTILITY

Infection

Pelvic inflammatory disease (PID) is a major cause of infertility. Complete blockage of the distal end of the Fallopian tube may result as a consequence of PID. Pelvic inflammatory disease is caused by sexually transmitted diseases, or following miscarriage, termination of pregnancy, surgical procedures involving uterine cavity, puerperal sepsis, or insertion of intrauterine contraceptive device. The severity of tubal factor infertility following PID is associated with the frequency and severity of PID episodes.[7]

Infection by chlamydia trachomatis is the most common sexually transmitted disease in the United Kingdom.[8] In a Scandinavian study, approximately 40 percent of all genital infections in women were complicated by an ascending infection and had signs of PID. Chlamydia infections may be asymptomatic or have very few signs of infection. Both symptomatic and asymptomatic chlamydial infections can damage the reproductive tract by inducing cell-mediated immune reactions leading to loss of tubal mucociliary cell activity as well as fibrosis and scarring resulting in tubal obliteration.[9] Rates of chlamydial infection continue to rise as a consequence of its asymptomatic nature.[8]

Neisseria gonorrhoeae infections are particularly common in young, urban women of low socioeconomic background and in those with multiple sexual partners.[10] The urogenital tract is most frequently infected because of the organism's predilection for columnar or pseudostratified epithelium.[11] Retrospective studies have shown that more than 60 percent of women with prior gonococcal infection have tubal factor infertility.[12] Gonorrhea may present as a localized infection of the lower genital tract, as an invasive infection of the upper genital tract, or as disseminated disease with systemic manifestations.

Pelvic tuberculosis is a frequent cause of PID and infertility in non-Western parts of the world. In India, women with a history of genital tuberculosis were found to have a rate of infertility of 58 percent. Tubal factor infertility was considered the cause of infertility in 41 percent of the women studied.[13] Genital tuberculosis can cause simple tubal blockage, tubo-ovarian abscess, or dense pelvic adhesions.

Bacterial vaginosis is a clinical syndrome caused by a shift in the vaginal flora from a predominance of *Lactobacillus* flora to one characterized by high concentrations of *Gardnerella vaginalis*, *Mycoplasma hominis*, and anaerobic bacteria.[14] Bacterial vaginosis has been shown to be present in 61 percent of patients with acute salpingitis, and bacterial vaginosis microorganisms are commonly isolated from the upper genital tracts of patients with PID.[15]

Pelvic infection secondary to actinomyces is a complication of intrauterine contraceptive device. Although rare, pelvic actinomycosis is a potentially life-threatening and fertility-destroying condition.[16] Other microorganisms have been found in patients with PID. These include *Escherichia* coli and other enteric organisms, organisms found in the abnormal vaginal flora of women with bacterial vaginosis, as well as *Mycoplasma hominis* and *Ureaplasma urealyticum.*

Endometriosis

Endometriosis is a common, benign, estrogen-dependent, chronic gynecological disorder associated with infertility. Patients with endometriosis have been shown to have a significant reduction in physiologic uterotubal sperm transport capacity.[17] Infertility in pelvic endometriosis is most probably caused by tubal distortion and limitation of fimbrial mobility due to associated pelvic adhesions.[10]

Surgery

History of pelvic surgery is a recognized risk factor for tubal infertility.[18] Pelvic surgery can lead to adhesion formation and tubal obstruction due to the close proximity of the Fallopian tubes to the surgical area. Surgical intervention for the management of tubal ectopic pregnancy leads to either salpingectomy or salpingostomy. Female sterilization involves intentional destruction of tubal patency. Previous history of other intra-abdominal operations such as bowel resection or urological procedures may also lead to peritubal adhesions.

OTHER CAUSES

Proximal tubal obstruction may result from salpingitis isthmica nodosa (SIN). SIN is defined as the microscopic presence of tubal epithelium within a hypertrophied and hyperplastic myosalpinx or beneath the tubal serosa, and characterized radiologically by a small diverticulum.[19] Other causes include cornual polyps if bilateral. Congenital abnormalities affect up to 10 percent of females and can affect the Fallopian tubes. The congenital abnormality includes the proximal isthmic portion or the proximal ampullary segment, and is especially associated with uterine anomalies.[20–22] Tubal obstruction may also result from an altered immunochemical and hormonal environment such as in the formation of keloid scars with altered fibroproliferation, producing significant deformations and altered organ function.[23]

TUBAL DISEASE AND IVF OUTCOME

Historically, in vitro fertilization-embryo transfer (IVF-ET) was developed to establish pregnancy in patients with tubal factor infertility.[24] The underlying principle for IVF-ET is that in the presence of abnormally functioning Fallopian tubes, an effective approach to treatment would be to bypass the contribution of these structures to the reproductive process. However, studies have reported that in a subset of patients with tubal disease due to hydrosalpinges, these patients have decreased IVF-ET pregnancy and delivery rates.[25–28] It is ironic that many women who have Fallopian tube disease, the very condition that IVF was designed to treat, actually have a reduced likelihood of successful pregnancy. It has been demonstrated that for patients having IVF-ET, the presence of a hydrosalpinges adversely affects the pregnancy rate, implantation rate, the live delivery rate per transfer, and the rate of early pregnancy loss in comparison to women with tubal damage but without hydrosalpinges.[29] There are suggestions that the milder forms of tubal disease, where no hydrosalpinx is present, may not have a negative impact on the likelihood of pregnancy from IVF treatment,[30] and those patients with tubal disease have cumulative conception and live-birthrates comparable to those with other causes of infertility.[31] Furthermore, when the distinction is made between unilateral and bilateral hydrosalpinx, the pregnancy and implantation rates are significantly higher among patients with unilateral hydrosalpinx.[32] The harmful effect of hydrosalpinx on the development of a pregnancy after IVF may thus have a threshold effect, and this threshold of toxicity may be reached much more frequently in cases of bilateral hydrosalpinges.[29]

Various pathophysiological hypotheses have been suggested to explain the lower pregnancy rates in the presence of hydrosalpinges. A permanent communication between the tube and the uterine cavity allows the passage of tubal fluid into the uterine cavity.[25,33] The flow of fluid may hinder the implantation of the embryo mechanically by flushing the uterine cavity. Fluid in the hydrosalpinx contains lower levels of proteins and bicarbonate than serum does, and may also contain cellular or infectious debris, lymphocytes, and other components, which may include cytokines, prostaglandins, leukotrienes, and catecholamines, all of which may have deleterious inflammatory, infectious, or immunological effects.[29] These components may have deleterious effects on the embryo or endometrium.[34]

Due to the evidence of hydrosalpinges compromising pregnancy in IVF-ET patients, some authorities are advising salpingectomy prior to IVF-ET. Studies have shown that performing salpingectomy or bipolar cauterization to proximally occlude the hydrosalpinx has been shown to improve pregnancy rates over control groups that have not undergone these prophylactic procedures.[34–38] Alternative prophylactic procedures suggested include hysteroscopic placement of a microinsert to proximally occlude the hydrosalpinx.[39] Hysteroscopic placement of a microinsert into the uterotubal junction is a recently introduced, non-incisional approach for permanent sterilization.

However, at the present time, due to the small number of randomized control trials with regards to occlusion or removal of hydrosalpinges prior to IVF-ET, it should remain only a consideration until universal agreement is achieved. This is because performing salpingectomy will involve a surgery and its associated risk.

EFFECT OF SURGERY ON OVARIAN RESPONSE DURING IVF

Aside from general surgical risk associated with laparoscopy or laparotomy for salpingectomy such as bleeding, infection, and internal organ injury, the effect of salpingectomy on ovarian function is uncertain and remains a matter of debate. The mechanism by which salpingectomy may negatively affect the ovarian response is not fully understood. The close anatomical association of the vascular and nervous supply to the Fallopian tubes and ovaries constitutes the rationale for the risk of impaired ovarian function following surgery. There are mixed reports regarding this issue. Some studies have shown a decreased response in the ovary ipsilateral to the site of salpingectomy, although there was no detrimental effect on the total ovarian response during IVF-ET.[40] Another study has shown a decrease in the total ovarian response following salpingectomy,[41] while some have shown no significant differences in the response to ovarian stimulation before and after salpingectomy.[42] Until a large prospective randomized control trial is conducted, caution should be exercised, especially in women whose second ovary is already compromised or missing.

EFFECT OF TUBAL DISEASE ON ENDOMETRIUM AND IMPLANTATION

There are various causes that could impair the embryo implantation in patients with tubal factor infertility. As mentioned previously, the reflux of hydrosalpinges fluid into the uterine cavity from the Fallopian tubes could produce a mechanical flushing effect that inhibits implantation.[33] Fluid in the uterine cavity during implantation may also exert a direct detrimental effect. The presence of a small amount of fluid in the endometrial cavity may interfere with the implantation process, as the pinopodes on the luminal surface of the endometrial epithelial cells may have the function of extracting fluid from the microenvironment of the embryo, thus facilitating its contact with the endometrium during implantation.[43] Steroids are thought to affect secretions in the Fallopian tubes and uterine cavity. Alterations in their levels and/or receptor expression could contribute to a poor uterine environment. The pinopodes on the luminal surface could be influenced by progesterone.[44] Their malfunction under altered progesterone levels would leave the transferred blastocysts stranded in a mass of uterine fluid.[45] Furthermore, in IVF-ET cycle, Sharara and McClamrock showed reflux of hydrosalpinges fluid into the endometrium following the administration of human chorionic gonadotropin (hCG [46]).

Endometrium could be damaged simultaneously with the acute phase damage of the Fallopian tubes, resulting in diminished capacity for embryo implantation.[26] It has also been suggested that chronic endometritis because of chlamydia or the effect of protein expression might directly affect endometrial receptivity.[47] Cells infected with *Chlamydia trachomatis* may produce a reduced amount of major structural proteins. Epithelial cell exfoliation, thinning and transformation from columnar to flat cuboidal epithelium in a hydrosalpinx, may reduce the apically located CFTR that regulates vesicular trafficking of epithelial cell-synthesized sulphated glycoproteins. Those are essential for early embryo development.[45] Bioactive substances such as tumor necrosis factor and other growth hormones associated with salpingitis have been shown to alter both endometrial stromal and epithelial cells.[48]

IVF STIMULATION REGIMENS FOR THE PATIENTS WITH TUBAL DISEASE

IVF stimulation regimens for the recruitment of multiple fertilizable oocytes have been constantly evolving and refined over the last 25 years. The overall aim is to achieve a satisfactory yield of mature oocytes without risking ovarian hyperstimulation. Traditionally, ovarian stimulation has been achieved using human menopausal gonadotrophin or purified urinary follicle stimulation hormone (FSH). More recently, recombinant gonadotrophins (r-FSH and r-LH) have become available. A systematic review has shown that urinary and recombinant gonadotropins are equally safe and effective.[49] Pituitary downregulation using GnRH analogues is often employed during ovarian stimulation to suppress endogenous luteinizing hormone and minimize the risk of a premature LH surge. It also allows for greater flexibility in timing and scheduling of treatment. Pituitary downregulation is achieved using either GnRH agonists or antagonists. For several years, GnRH agonists were the only GnRH analogue available for pituitary downregulation. Despite the fact that the use of GnRH agonists was associated with several disadvantages, they were uniformly accepted in ovarian stimulation for IVF because they increased pregnancy rates when compared with cycles without downregulation.[50] GnRH antagonists provide several advantages over GnRH agonists in terms of fewer injections, fewer treatment days, and avoidance of the adverse effects of agonists, which include cyst formation and signs and symptoms of estrogen deprivation.[49] From the prospective of live birth outcome, there is no significant difference between the two GnRH analogues used.[51]

For patients having IVF due to tubal factor, there are currently no published data comparing the different IVF protocols and its outcome. Therefore, the optimal stimulation regime for patients with tubal factor infertility would be the one that maximizes the recruitment of fertilizable oocytes and minimizes the adverse risks such as ovarian hyperstimulation syndrome.

OOCYTE COLLECTION AND HYDROSALPINX

Tubo-ovarian abscess and febrile morbidity is a rare but potentially serious complication following in vitro fertilization and embryo transfer. The potential for inadvertent introduction of aspiration needle into the hydrosalpinx during oocyte retrieval is high as the ultrasonic appearance may look similar to a follicle to the unwary. Although there is no randomized controlled trial published, there have been numerous case reports of tubo-ovarian abscess following IVF treatment. However, not all are related to hydrosalpinx.[52–56] Majority of cases occurred within days of the procedures, while some occurred several weeks following the initial oocyte retrieval.[52,54] Possible explanation for the development of tubo-ovarian abscess is the activation of quiescent bacteria within the Fallopian tubes from previous pelvic infection that caused the tubal infertility.[53,55] Hence, the administration of prophylactic broad spectrum antibiotics is recommended if the hydrosalpinx is aspirated, either intentionally or inadvertently.[53]

SUCCESS RATES FOLLOWING TUBAL FACTOR IVF AT VARIOUS AGES

Meta-analysis by Camus et al. showed pregnancy rates to be significantly lower in the presence of hydrosalpinx. The pregnancy rates were 31.2 percent in the group of patients with tubal factor infertility without hydrosalpinx compared to

19.7 percent with hydrosalpinx. Similarly, the delivery rate per transfer in the group without hydrosalpinx was 23.4 percent and in the group with hydrosalpinx was 13.4 percent.[29] In another study by Strandell et al., cumulative results of IVF were obtained following salpingectomy on patients with hydrosalpinx. This study found that the implantation rate was significantly higher in patients who had salpingectomy (27.2%) compared to ones who did not have salpingectomy (20.2%).[57]

There are many factors that can affect the success rates in IVF. These include the patient's age, past reproductive history, quality of ovarian stimulation, the quality and number of embryos transferred, and number of previous treatment cycles. Age of women is well known to be the most important factor affecting fertility treatment and particularly in IVF treatment.[58] A study by Check et al. comparing the cumulative probability of pregnancy after IVF by age and tubal factor infertility found that the 3-month cumulative probability of pregnancy based on life table analysis was 33 percent in women under age 35 and 25 percent in women over age 35.[59]

SUMMARY

In vitro fertilization was first pioneered by Steptoe and Edwards in 1978 to overcome tubal factor infertility. It is ironic that the very condition that IVF was pioneered to treat actually reduces the likelihood of successful outcome. The delivery of cost-effective treatment for tubal factor infertility that is evidence based is a difficult task, given the limited availability of well-designed randomized controlled trials and variation in patients' expectations, values, and beliefs. Patients with tubal factor infertility should be counseled fully about the success and cost-effectiveness of assisted conception technique prior to commencing treatment, with special emphasis on age factor.

REFERENCES

1. Diaz S, Ortiz M, Crozatto H. Studies on the duration of ovum transport by the human oviduct. The time interval between the luteinizing hormone peak and recovery of ova by transcervical flushing of the uterus in normal woman. *Am J Obstet Gynecol.* 1980;**137**:116.
2. Lippes J, Enders R, Pragay D, Bartholomew W. The collection and analysis of human Fallopian tube fluid. *Contraception.* 1973;**5**:85–93.
3. Macmillan S. Tubal factor infertility. In: Milton P, editor. *Management of infertility for the MRCOG and beyond.* Place: RCOG Press; 2000. pp. 71–86.
4. Serafini P, Batzofin J. Diagnosis of female infertility. A comprehensive approach. *J Reprod Med.* 1989;**34**(1):29–40.
5. Bahamondes L, Bueno J, Hardy E, Vera S, Pimentel E, Ramos M. Identification of main risk factors for tubal infertility. *Fertil Steril.* 1994;**61**(3):478–82.
6. DeCherney A. Anything you can do I can do better or differently! *Fertil Steril.* 1987;**48**: 374–6.
7. Weström L, Joesoef R, Reynolds G, Hagdu A, Thompson S. Pelvic inflammatory disease and fertility. A cohort study of 1,844 women with laparoscopically verified disease and

657 control women with normal laparoscopic results. *Sex Trans Dis.* 1992;**19**(4):185–92.
8. Chief Medical Officer's Medical Advisory Group. Main Report of the CMO's Expert Advisory Group on Chlamydia trachomatis. London: Department of Health; 1998.
9. Mardh P-A. Tubal factor infertility, with special regard to chlamydial salpingitis. *Curr Opin Infect Dis.* 2004;**17**(1):49–52.
10. Khalaf Y. Tubal subfertility. *BMJ.* 2003;**327**(7415):610–13.
11. Rhoton-Vlasak A. Infections and infertility. *Prim Care Update Ob Gyns.* 2000;**7**(5):200.
12. Wiesenfeld HC, Hillier SL, Krohn MA, Amortegui AJ, Heine RP, Landers DV, Sweet RL. Lower genital tract infection and endometritis: insight into subclinical pelvic inflammatory disease. *Obstet Gynecol.* 2002;**100**(3):456.
13. Tripathy SN, Tripathy SN. Infertility and pregnancy outcome in female genital tuberculosis. *Int J Gynecol Obstet.* 2002;**76**(2):159.
14. Hillier SL, Kiviat NB, Hawes SE, Hasselquist MB, Hanssen PW, Eschenbach DA, Holmes KK. Role of bacterial vaginosis-associated microorganisms in endometritis. *Am J Obstet Gynecol.* 1996;**175**(2):435.
15. Soper DE, Brockwell NJ, Dalton HP, Johnson D. Observations concerning the microbial etiology of acute salpingitis. *Am J Obstet Gynecol.* 1994;**170**(4):1008.
16. Guillebaud J. *Contraception today*, 5th ed. Place: Martin Dunitz; 2004.
17. Kissler S, Zangos S, Wiegratz I, Kohl J, Rody A, Gaetje R, Doebert N, Wildt L, Kunz G, Leyendecker G, Kaufmann M. Utero-tubal sperm transport and its impairment in endometriosis and adenomyosis. *Ann NY Acad Sci.* 2007;**1101**:38–48.
18. Bahamondes L, Bueno JG, Hardy E, Vera S, Pimentel E, Ramos M. Identification of main risk factors for tubal infertility. *Fertil Steril.* 1994;**61**(3):478–82.
19. Margara R, Trew G. Tubal disease. In: Shaw R, Soutter W, Stanton S, editors. *Gynaecology.* Place: Churchill Livingstone; 1997. pp. 319–28.
20. Nawroth F, Nugent W, Ludwig M. Congenital partial atresia of the Fallopian tube. *Reprod Biomed Online.* 2006;**12**(2):205–8.
21. Johnston A, McComb P. Fertility potential of women with congenital ampullary atresia of the Fallopian tube. *Fertil Steril.* 2003;**79**(2):431–3.
22. Dahan M, Burney R, Lathi R. Congenital interruption of the ampullary portion of the Fallopian tube. *Fertil Steril.* 2006;**85**(6):1820–1.
23. Garcia-Ulloa A, Arrieta O. Tubal occlusion causing infertility due to an excessive inflammatory response in patients with predisposition for keloid formation. *Med Hypotheses.* 2005;**65**(5):908–14.
24. Steptoe PC, Edwards RG. Birth after reimplantation of human embryo. *Lancet.* 1978;**2**(8085):366.
25. Chien L-W, Au H-K, Xiao J, Tzeng C-R. Fluid accumulation within the uterine cavity reduces pregnancy rates in women undergoing IVF. *Hum Reprod.* 2002;**17**(2):351–6.
26. Strandell A, Waldenstrom U, Nilsson L, Hamberger L. Hydrosalpinx reduces in-vitro fertilization/embryo transfer pregnancy rates. *Hum Reprod.* 1994;**9**(5):861–3.
27. Andersen AN, Yue Z, Meng FJ, Petersen K. Implantation: low implantation rate after in-vitro fertilization in patients with hydrosalpinges diagnosed by ultrasonography. *Hum Reprod.* 1994;**9**(10):1935–8.
28. Vandromme J, Chasse E, Lejeune B, Van Rysselberge M, Delvigne A, Leroy F. Infertility: hydrosalpinges in in-vitro fertilization: an unfavourable prognostic feature. *Hum Reprod.* 1995;**10**(3):576–9.
29. Camus E, Poncelet C, Goffinet F, Wainer B, Merlet F, Nisand I, Philippe HJ. Pregnancy rates after in-vitro fertilization in cases of tubal infertility with and without hydrosalpinx: a meta-analysis of published comparative studies. *Hum Reprod.* 1999;**14**(5):1243–9.
30. Johnson N, Sadler L, Merrilees M. IVF and tubal pathology – not all bad news. *Aust NZ J Obstet Gynaecol.* 2002;**42**(3):285–8.
31. Tan SL, Royston P, Campbell S, Jacobs HS, Betts J, Mason BA, Edwards RG. Cumulative conception and live birth rates after in-vitro fertilisation. *Lancet*, 1992;**339**:1390–4.

32. Wainer B, Camus E, Camier B. Does hydrosalpinges reduce the pregnancy rate following in vitro fertilisation? *Fertil Steril.* 1997;**68**:1022–6.
33. Mansour R, Aboulghar M, Serour G, Riad R. Fluid accumulation of the uterine cavity before embryo transfer: a possible hindrance for implantation. *J In Vitro Fert Embryo Transf.* 1991;**8**(3):157–9.
34. Murray CA, Clarke HJ, Tulandi T, Tan SL. Inhibitory effect of human hydrosalpingeal fluid on mouse preimplantation embryonic development is significantly reduced by the addition of lactate. *Human Reproduction,* 1997;**12**:2504–7.
35. Dechaud H, Anahory T, Aligier N, Arnal F, Humeau H, Hedon B. Salpingectomy for repeated embryo nonimplantation after in vitro fertilisation in patients with severe tubal factor infertility. *J Assist Reprod Genet.* 2000;**17**(4):200–6.
36. Dechaud H, Daures J, Arnal F, Humeau H, Hedon B. Does previous salpingectomy improve implantation and pregnancy rates in patients with severe tubal factor infertility who are undergoing in vitro fertilisation? A pilot prospective randomised study. *Fertil Steril.* 1998;**69**(6):1020–5.
37. Johnson N, Mak W, Sowter M. Laparoscopic salpingectomy for women with hydrosalpinges enhances the success of IVF: a Cochrane review. *Hum Reprod.* 2002;**17**(3): 543–8.
38. Murray D, Sagoskin A, Widra E, Levy M. The adverse effect of hydrosalpinges on in vitro fertilisation pregnancy rates and the benefit of surgical correction. *Fertil Steril.* 1998;**69**(1):41–5.
39. Rosenfield R, Stones R, Coates A, Matteri R, Hesla J. Proximal occlusion of hydrosalpinx by hysteroscopic placement of microinsert before in vitro fertlilisation-embryo transfer. *Fertil Steril.* 2005;**83**(5):1547.e11–e14.
40. Lass A, Ellenbogen A, Croucher C, Trew G, Margara R, Becattini C, Winston R. Effect of salpingectomy on ovarian response to superovulation in an in vitro fertilization-embryo transfer program. *Fertil Steril.* 1998;**70**(6):1035–8.
41. Gelbaya TA, Nardo LG, Fitzgerald CT, Horne G, Brison DR, Lieberman BA. Ovarian response to gonadotropins after laparoscopic salpingectomy or the division of Fallopian tubes for hydrosalpinges. *Fertil Steril.* 2006;**85**(5):1464–8.
42. Starandell A, Lindhard A, Waldenstrom U, Thorburn J. Prophylactic salpingectomy does not impair the ovarian response in IVF treatment. *Hum Reprod.* 2001;**16**:1135–9.
43. Edwards R. Why are agonadal and post-amenorrhoeic women so fertile after oocyte donation? *Hum Reprod.* 1992;**7**:733–4.
44. Martel D, Monier MN, Roche D, Psychoyos A. Hormonal dependence of pinopode formation at the uterine luminal surface. *Hum Reprod.* 1991;**6**(4):597–603.
45. Ajonuma LC, Ng EHY, Chan HC. New insights into the mechanisms underlying hydrosalpinx fluid formation and its adverse effect on IVF outcome. *Hum Reprod Update.* 2002;**8**(3):255–64.
46. Sharara FI, McClamrock HD. Endometrial fluid collection in women with hydrosalpinx after human chorionic gonadotrophin administration: a report of two cases and implications for management. *Hum Reprod.* 1997;**12**(12):2816–19.
47. Sharara F, Scott R, Marut E, Queenan J. In vitro fertilisation outcome in women with hydrosalpinx. *Hum Reprod.* 1996;**11**:526–30.
48. Toth M, Jeremias J, Ledger W, Witkins S. In vivo tumour necrosis factor reproduction in women with salpingitis. *Surg Gynecol Obstet.* 1992;**174**:359–62.
49. Muasher S, Abdallah R, Hubayter Z. Optimal stimulation protocols for in vitro fertilization. *Fertil Steril.* 2006;**86**(2):267–73.
50. Tarlatzis BC, Kolibianakis EM. GnRH agonists vs antagonists. *Best Pract Res Clin Obstet Gynaecol.* 2007;**21**(1):57–65.
51. Kolibianakis EM, Collins J, Tarlatzis BC, Devroey P, Diedrich K, Griesinger G. Among patients treated for IVF with gonadotropins and GnRH analogues, is the probability of live birth dependent on the type of analogue used? A systematic review and meta-analysis. *Hum Reprod Update.* 2006;**12**(6):651–71.

52. Sharpe K, Karovitch AJ, Claman P, Suh KN. Transvaginal oocyte retrieval for in vitro fertilization complicated by ovarian abscess during pregnancy. *Fertil Steril.* 2006;**86**(1): 219.
53. Peters A, Hecht B, Durinzi K, DeLeon F, Wentz A. Salpingitis or oophoritis: what causes fever following oocyte aspiration and embryo transfer? *Obstet Gynecol.* 1993;**81**(5(Pt 2)):876–7.
54. Matsunaga Y, Fukushima K, Nozaki M, Nakanami N, Kawano Y, Shigematsu T, Satoh S, Nakano H. A case of pregnancy complicated by the development of a tubo-ovarian abscess following in vitro fertilization and embryo transfer. *Am J Perinatol.* 2003;**20**(6):277–82.
55. Varras M, Polyzos D, Tsikini A, Antypa E, Apessou D, Tsouroulas M. Ruptured tubo-ovarian abscess as a complication of IVF treatment: clinical, ultrasonographic, and histopathologic findings. A case report. *Clin Exp Obstet Gynecol.* 2003;**30**(2–3):164–8.
56. Coccia ME, Cammilli F, Ginocchioni L, Rizzello F. Role of infection in in vitro fertilization treatment. *Ann NY Acad Sci.* 2004;**1034**(1):219–35.
57. Strandell A, Lindhard A, Waldenstrom U, Thorburn J. Hydrosalpinx and IVF outcome: cumulative results after salpingectomy in a randomized controlled trial. *Hum Reprod.* 2001;**16**(11):2403–10.
58. Templeton A, Morris JK, Parslow W. Factors that affect outcome of in-vitro fertilisation treatment. *Lancet.* 1996;**348**(9039):1402–6.
59. Check J, Lurie D, Callan C, Baker A, Benfer K. Comparison of the cumulative probability of pregnancy after in vitro fertilization-embryo transfer by infertility factor and age. *Fertil Steril.* 1994;**61**(2):257–61.

X

TUBAL STERILIZATION

Hany Lashen

INTRODUCTION

Tubal occlusion has increasingly become a popular method of contraception so that 22 percent and 11 percent of women in the developed and developing world, respectively, are reported to have been sterilized in 1990.[1] These women represented 44 percent and 18 percent of all contraceptive users, respectively. As of 2003, more than two hundred million women of reproductive age were sterilized worldwide.[2] In a study of the General Practice Research Database, it was suggested that in 1999 an estimated 47,268 tubal occlusions and 64,422 vasectomies were performed in England in the National Health Service and charitable sectors.

The increase in tubal sterilization in the United States was more noticeable from the 1970s onwards when the number of procedures of bilateral tubal occlusion or destruction of the Fallopian tubes increased from 201,000 in 1970 to a peak of 702,000 by 1977.[3] The exact reason for the surge in tubal sterilization is not entirely known; however, several factors may have contributed. Increasing safety of anesthesia and surgical procedures and the introduction of laparoscopic surgery that entailed a shorter hospital stay and quicker postoperative recovery are in the forefront of all the potential reasons. From the patients' point of view, the concern about the safety of long-term use of the available contraceptive methods such as the combined oral contraceptive (COC) pill and intrauterine contraceptive devices (IUCD) would have certainly contributed to the sharp rise in the use of female sterilization. Permanent methods of contraception generally and female sterilization particularly have been the subject of ethical debate even when the request for sterilization is voluntary. Recent debate over involuntary sterilization of mentally handicapped young adults has received media attention. In this chapter, ethical issues surrounding female sterilization will not be covered unless it has a pertinent clinical significance.

RATIONALE AND OBJECTIVES

The rationale and objective of female sterilization is best described through the statement of the World Health Organization Task Force on female sterilization:[4] "The ideal female sterilization would involve a simple, easily learned, one-time procedure that could be accomplished under local anesthesia and involve tubal occlusion technique that caused minimum damage. The procedure would be safe, have high efficacy, be readily accessible, and be personally and culturally acceptable. The cost for each procedure would be low and there would be minimal cost for maintenance of equipments."

There are no absolute contraindications; however, several issues need to be considered with regard to the consent and the implications counseling offered to patients. The Royal College of Obstetricians and Gynaecologists (RCOG[5]) in their clinical guidelines on male and female sterilization indicated that there were no absolute contraindications to sterilization of men or women, provided that they make the request themselves, are of sound mind, and are not acting under external duress. When seeing a woman requesting sterilization, a history should be taken and an examination should be carried out on every person requesting sterilization so that other problems of confounding issues can be identified and dealt with. Because of the long-term effect of the procedure and potential risk implications, counseling is mandatory, which should be provided within the context of a service offering a full range of information about and access to other long-term reversible methods of contraception. This should also include information on the advantages, disadvantages, and relative failure rates of each method.

If there is any question of a person not having the mental capacity to consent to a procedure that will permanently remove his or her fertility, Government guidelines make it clear that the case should be referred to court for judgment.

METHODS

Until the introduction of laparoscopy, tubal ligation via mini-laparotomy was the method of choice for female sterilization and most cases were carried out postcaesarean section. Laparoscopic sterilization was developed by Steptoe[6] and has been the preferred method of choice for obvious reasons ever since. Although the WHO Task Force[4] did not promote either laparoscopy or mini-laparotomy, it came close to endorsing that either procedure will be adequate provided the criteria described earlier were observed. In a systematic review, Kulier et al.[7] examined all the available literature on laparoscopic female sterilization and that carried out via mini-laparotomy. They concluded that major morbidities seemed to be a rare outcome for both laparoscopy and minilaparotomy. The studies they included in their analysis had limited power to demonstrate significant difference for the relatively rare but potentially serious outcome. The authors then advised against sterilization via culdoscopy due to the reported higher complications rate. This view was also shared by RCOG[5] in their evidence-based clinical guidelines on male and female sterilization. Personal preference of the clinician and the woman, as well as other practical aspects including the clinician's expertise, may determine which method is used.

More recently, hysteroscopic sterilization has been employed and is still under evaluation. Currently, only one method of hysteroscopic sterilization is licensed for use in the UK, which consists of a dynamically expanding metal micro-insert (Essure, Conceptus, SAS, France). Inserting the Essure into the Fallopian tube under hysteroscopic vision is relatively safe and easy enough to perform on an outpatient basis. The insert induces fibrosis, which occludes the tube. This needs to be confirmed 3 months later with a hysterosalpingogram during which time another form of contraception should be used.

Having discussed the access route generally, the tubal occlusion methods will now be discussed.

1. Pomeroy tubal ligation: In this operation, a knuckle of the Fallopian tube (ampullary portion) is pulled up with mosquito hemostat or Allis clamp. A small clamp is put across the base and the part in between is cut with scissors or knife. The remaining part of the tube is then sutured with any appropriate suture material. Although this procedure can be done through laparoscopy, it has traditionally been done via a mini-laparotomy, and the introduction of other laparoscopic procedures has made it redundant except for postcaesarean section.
2. Tubal fulguration with diathermy: Both monopolar and bipolar diathermy have been used to destroy the Fallopian tube. Several complications and accidents have been reported, including thermal injury to bowel[8] and skin,[9] face, and hand of operator, and death.[9] Tubal diathermy is no longer a common practice in female sterilization; however, it has a place in some cases where other methods have failed. It is noteworthy that the tubal destruction is more significant so that reversal is less successful. It has also been reported that ectopic pregnancy following tubal destruction with diathermy is more likely due to the formation of utero-peritoneal fistula.[10] The use of bipolar diathermy is safer than monopolar diathermy although it has a higher failure rate.
3. Tubal occlusion using Filshie clips, tubal rings, and Hulka-Clemens Spring Clip: These methods have been more popular because the tubal destruction is minimal. Compared to tubal diathermy, this is associated with less postoperative pain and has a better success rate when reversal of sterilization is carried out.
    a. Filshie clips: A clip made out of titanium and lined with silicon rubber. It is hinged so that it can lock over the tube. A special applicator is used that requires an 8-mm port to introduce into the abdomen. Approximately 4 mm of the tube is destroyed as a result of using these clips.[11]
    b. Silastic (Falope or Yoon) rings: Made essentially of nonreactive Silastic, these are rubber bands that has a 100 percent elastic memory if stretched to less than 6 mm for a brief time. They are introduced into the abdomen using a special applicator that is designed to grasp a loop of the tube and release the ring on it. This renders the approximately 2.5-cm loop avascular, which can be removed and sent for histology if need be. The use of this method is associated with a higher incidence of postoperative pain and has lower reversibility success rates.[11]
    c. Hulka-Clemens Spring Clip: Made of two plastic jaws made of Lexan and hinged by a small metal pin. Each jaw has teeth on the inside surface. When together, the jaws occlude approximately 3 mm of the tube.

4. Essure:[12] The Essure microinsert consists of a stainless steel inner coil, a nitinol, super-elastic outer coil, and polyethylene (PET) fibers. The PET fibers are wound in and around the inner coil. The microinsert is 4 cm in length and 0.8 mm in diameter in its wound-down configuration. When released, the outer coil expands to 1.5 to 2.0 mm to anchor the microinsert in the varied diameters and shapes of the Fallopian tube. It can be introduced in an office procedure or as a day case. The insert is introduced under hysteroscopic vision and the use of normal saline to distend the uterine cavity. Training is required to be able to insert the Essure effectively into the uterine tubes. Occasionally inserting the coil is not feasible even in experienced hands because of uterine malformation or tubal spasm.[13] Unlike tubal ligation, Essure is not immediately effective and tissue fibrosis is required that can take up to 12 weeks. A hysterosalpingogram is required at approximately 12 weeks to ensure tubal occlusion. Alternate contraceptive methods should be used until occlusion can be demonstrated.[14]

COMPLICATIONS

Regret

Female sterilization is intended as a permanent method of contraception and most of the women who are sterilized are happy with the outcome. However, approximately 3 to 10 percent of women later regret having been sterilized.[15] Curtis et al.[16] carried out a systematic review of all the studies that examined the effect of age on the incidence of regret in women who underwent sterilization. They reported that women who were age 30 or younger at the time of sterilization were twice as likely to experience regret. However, the most common reason for requesting reversal of sterilization or IVF was a new relationship.[17] Of course, the younger the woman, the more likely that a new relationship can result in a desire to have more children. As a precaution against the risk of later regret, additional care must be taken when counseling people under age 30 or people without children. Care should also be exercised in discussions with people making decisions during pregnancy, or in reaction to a loss of relationship, or who may be at risk of coercion by partners, family, or health or social welfare professionals. Counselors and advisers should also be aware and take account of cultural, religious, psychosocial, psychosexual, and other psychological issues because some of these may have implications beyond fertility.[5]

Procedure Failure

It is important to realize and inform the women that tubal occlusion is not a totally fail-safe procedure. The RCOG suggested using the term *tubal occlusion* instead of sterilization as the former is more factual. The risk of failure after sterilization is measured by the number of pregnancies that occur afterwards. There are two types of pregnancy: a luteal phase pregnancy (i.e., that which occurred immediately before the surgery) and pregnancies that occur subsequent to sterilization. The risk of the first is dependent on the timing of the procedure and the method of contraception used prior to it and has been excluded in all the published studies. However, the latter is primarily dependent on the method used and other technical factors such as the expertise of the operator. It has to be emphasized that the failure risk does not decline with time. Earlier studies underestimated the failure rate, which is more likely to be down to the short follow-up period due to the false assumption that most pregnancies take place shortly after surgery.

The mechanism through which tubal occlusion can fail would be:

a. Recanalization of the tubal ends
b. Utero-peritoneal fistula formation
c. Slipping of the occlusive devicc
d. Incomplete occlusion of the tube
e. Technical error, such as incorrectly placing or applying the occlusive device, which can also be due to equipment failure.

The failure rates vary according to the procedure and the length of followup in the reported longitudinal studies. The Collaborative Review of Sterilization (CREST) study that included 10,685 women for a long follow-up period reported a cumulative failure rate of 18.5 per 1,000 for all methods combined.[18] This was the only prospective large multicenter longitudinal study with long enough followup: 89 percent of all participants were interviewed in the first year, 81 percent at 3 years, 73 percent at 5 years, and 58 percent at 8–14 years. Despite the dropout rate toward the second half of the study, the number was large enough to provide an informative figure for the failure rate.

The analysis of the individual procedures showed that at 10 years, the most effective methods were salpingectomy and laparoscopic monopolar coagulation with a failure rate of 7.5/1,000. The Falope ring failure rate came second at 17.7/1,000, followed by interval partial salpingectomy at 20.1/1,000. The 10 years cumulative failure rates for bipolar coagulation and spring clips were 24.8/1,000 and 36.5/1,000, respectively. The CREST study reported that the pregnancy rate was influenced by the age of the woman at the time of sterilization and her ethnic origin, with more risk of failure among black and young women (women younger than age 28 were more likely to report failure than those older than age 34). They reported a relative risk of 2.53 for black women with a 95 percent CI of 1.59–4.02.

In the UK, most gynecologists use the Filshie clip.[19] As the Filshie clip was not included in the CREST study, most of the evidence to its efficacy is from smaller studies.[20–21] The RCOG suggested a crude 10-year failure rate of 2–3/1,000.[5]

Ectopic Pregnancy

Pregnancies occurring after sterilization are more likely to be ectopic.[22] Understandably, this carries a higher morbidity and mortality risk compared to intrauterine pregnancy. All women undergoing tubal occlusion should be counseled regarding this risk and advised that if pregnancy is suspected to seek medical advice. The incidence of ectopic pregnancy following tubal occlusion is procedure dependent and has been reported to range from 4.3 to 76 percent. Tubal occlusion using bipolar diathermy is associated with a higher risk of ectopic pregnancy as it is twenty-seven times likelier to lead to an ectopic pregnancy compared to partial salpingectomy.[23]

Menstrual Disturbances

Women who discontinue the oral contraceptive pills are likely to experience an increase in the menstrual blood flow. Accordingly, an ill-defined and controversial condition called "post-sterilization syndrome" was suggested. After much debate, it has been recognized that tubal occlusion is unlikely to lead to menstrual abnormalities.[24] In the CREST study, it was reported that women with menstrual dysfunction prior to sterilization were more likely to experience more changes afterwards and eventually have a hysterectomy.[18] In a study that was carried out in the United States, it was found that women with menstrual problems who were sterilized were more likely to be admitted to the hospital due to severe symptoms compared to those whose husbands had a vasectomy. It was also reported in the same study that the risk of admission to the hospital due to the severity of the symptoms was more likely if the patient was sterilized at a younger age.[25] A similar study in the UK reported that hospital referral due to menstrual disorders was no different between sterilized women and those whose husbands had a vasectomy.[26]

Long-Term Outcome

Two issues have been addressed with regard to the long-term outcome of tubal occlusion: hysterectomy and ovarian/breast cancer.

Hysterectomy

Several prospective studies addressed the risk of hysterectomy among women who underwent sterilization. Two cohort studies from the United States found that in women receiving care in the same health care system, those who were sterilized were more likely to have a hysterectomy.[27–28] In Canada and the UK where hysterectomy is less common compared to the United States, the picture was somehow different. In Canada, a cohort study found no overall increase in the risk of hysterectomy.[29] However, they reported a modest increase in the hysterectomy risk among the women who were sterilized at age 25–29 (RR = 1.6). In the UK, no overall increase in the risk of hysterectomy was found among sterilized women and no analysis per age was provided.[26] The contradiction in the studies' outcome may be due to several factors including the population studied, their views on surgery generally, and on hysterectomy, and the length of followup.

Ovarian and Breast Cancer

Recent studies have suggested a decreased risk of ovarian cancer among sterilized women.[30–31] These studies are among several that consistently described lower risk of ovarian cancer among sterilized women. However, not every study had enough information about potential confounding variables. The exact mechanism is not known and there has been speculation about occlusion preventing passage of ascending carcinogens, which is rather flimsy. With regard to breast cancer, one study showed association between tubal occlusion and breast cancer that was reassuring despite no other confirmation.[32] However, it was reported that women get less opportunity for screening if they were not on the oral contraceptive pill, which may cast some doubt on the validity of such studies.[33]

Reversal of Sterilization

When women are counseled about sterilization, they are always advised that the procedure is potentially irreversible. Regardless of this and the quality of counseling offered, request for reversals is inevitable. Up to 26 percent of women regretted being sterilized;[34] however, only a proportion of these women request reversal of sterilization. Here the success of reversal is briefly described.

Tubal reanastomosis gives a good chance of successful intrauterine pregnancy in up to 92 percent of cases.[5] This no doubt compares favorably with IVF. However, the risk of ectopic pregnancy is higher among patients undergoing tubal reanastomosis. The success of tubal reanastomosis is dependent on several factors including the tubal occlusion procedure and the woman's age. Women older than age 40 were reported to have a good success rate after reversal of sterilization.[35–36] Although the efficacy of IVF versus tubal reanastomosis has never been compared in a prospective randomized trial, the success rate from IVF in patients with tubal disease after age 40 is significantly low. The partner's semen parameters and the woman's ovulatory status are to be taken into account when considering the options.

REFERENCES

1. Peterson H, Pollack AE, Warshaw JS. Tubal sterilisation. In: Rock JA, Jones III HW, editors. *Te Linde's Operative Gynaecology*, 9th edition. Philadelphia: Lippincott Williams and Wilkins; 2003. pp. 537–56.
2. *United Nations. World contraceptive use*, 2003. New York: United Nations; 2005. http://www.un.org/esa/population/publications/contraceptive2003/WallChart˙CP2003.pdf.
3. Westhoff C, Davis A. Tubal sterilisation: a focus on the US experience. *Fertil Steril.* 2000;**73**:913–22.
4. WHO B 1982 (published data only). World Health Organisation. Task Force on Female Sterilisation. Special Programme of Research, Development, and Research Training in Human Reproduction. Mini-laparotomy or laparoscopy for sterilization. *Am J Obstet Gynaecol.* 1982;**143**:645–52.
5. National evidence-based clinical guidelines. Male and female sterilisation. 2004. http://www.rcog.org.uk/files/rcog-corp/uploaded-files/NEBSterilisationFull060607.pdf.
6. Steptoe PC. Recent advances in laparoscopic methods of control of fertility and infertility. *Br Med Bull.* 1970;**26**:60–4.
7. Kulier R, Boulvain M, De Candolle G, Campana A. Mini-laparotomy and endoscopic techniques for tubal sterilisation. *Cochrane Database of Systematic Reviews.* 2004;Issue 3. No.: CD001328. DOI: 10.1002/14651858.CD001328.pub2.

8. Maudsley RF, Qizilbash AH. Thermal injury to the bowel as a complication of laparoscopic sterilization. *Can J Surg.* 1979;**22**:232–4.
9. Corson SL, Patrick H, Hamilton T, Bolognese RJ. Electrical considerations of laparoscopic sterilization. *J Reprod Med.* 1973;**11**:159–64.
10. Phillips JM, Hulka B, Hulka JF, Keith D, Keith L. Laparoscopic procedures: the American Association of Gynecologic Laparoscopists' membership survey for 1975. *J Reprod Med.* 1977;18:227–32.
11. Wahab M, Li TC, Cooke ID. Reversal of sterilisation versus IVF: a cost-benefit analysis. *J Obstet Gynaecol.* 1997;17:180–5.
12. http://www.essure.co.uk/Home/WhatisEssure/tabid/138/Default.aspx (accessed September 2009).
13. Abbott J. Transvaginal sterilisation. *Best Pract Res Clin Obstet Gynaecol.* 2005;**19**:743–56.
14. Teoh M, Meagher S, Kovacs G. Ultrasound detection of the Essure permanent birth control device: a case series. *Aust N Z J Obstet Gynaecol.* 2003;43:378–80.
15. Wilcox LS, Chu SY, Eaker ED, Zeger SL, Peterson HB. Risk factors for regret after tubal sterilization: 5 years of follow-up in a prospective study. *Fertil Steril.* 1991;**55**:927–33.
16. Curtis KM, Mohllajee AP, Peterson HB. Regret following female sterilisation at a young age: a systematic review. *Contraception.* 2006;**73**:205–10.
17. Leader A, Galan N, George R, Taylor PJ. A comparison of definable traits in women requesting reversal of sterilization and women satisfied with sterilization. *Am J Obstet Gynecol.* 1983;**145**:198–202.
18. Peterson HB, Xia Z, Hughes JM, Wilcox LS, Tylor LR, Trussell J. The risk of pregnancy after tubal sterilization: findings from the U.S. Collaborative Review of Sterilization. *Am J Obstet Gynecol.* 1996;**174**:1161–8.
19. Garrud P, Sheard C, Filshie M, Beattie A. Elective female sterilisation: a survey of UK gynaecologists' practices. *CME Bull Gynaecol.* 2000;**2**:13–17.
20. Filshie GM, Helson K, Teper S. Day case sterilization with the Filshie Clip in Nottingham. 10-year follow-up study: the first 200 cases. In: Kruger T, Gome V, Van der Wat J, editors. 7th Annual Meeting of the International Society for Gynecologic Endoscopy. Bologna: Monduzzi Editore International Proceedings Division; 1998. pp. 145–58.
21. Kovacs GT, Krins AJ. Female sterilisations with Filshie clips: what is the risk failure? A retrospective survey of 30,000 applications. *J Fam Plann Reprod Health Care.* 2001;**28**:34–5.
22. Kjer JJ, Knudsen LB. Ectopic pregnancy subsequent to laparoscopic sterilisation. *Am J Obstet Gynaecol.* 1989;**160**:1202–4.
23. Peterson HB, Xia Z, Hughes JM, Wilcox LS, Tylor LR, Trussell J. The risk of ectopic pregnancy after tubal sterilization. *N Engl J Med.* 1997;**336**:762–7.
24. Rulin M, Davidson A, Philiber S, Graves W, Cushman W. Long-term effect of tubal sterilisation on menstrual disorders. *Obstet Gynaecol.* 19993;**82**:118–21.
25. Shy K, Stergachis A, Grothaus L, Wangner E, Hecht J, Anderson G. Tubal sterilisation and risk of subsequent hospital admission for menstrual disorders. *Am J Obstet Gynaecol.* 1992;**166**:1689–1702.
26. Vessey M, Huggies G, Lawless M, Yates D. Tubal sterilisation: findings in a large prospective study. *Br J Obstet Gynaecol.* 1993;**60**:203–9.
27. Stergachis A, Shy K, Grothaus L. Tubal sterilisation and the long-term risk of hysterectomy. *JAMA.* 1990;**264**:2893–8.
28. Goldhaber M, Armstrong M, Golditch I, Sheehe P, Petitti D. Griedman G. Long-term risk of hysterectomy among 80,007 sterilized and comparison women at Kaiser Permanente, 1971–78. *Am J Epidemiol.* 1993;**138**:508–21.
29. Cohn M. Long-term risk of hysterectomy after tubal sterilization. *Am J Epidemiol.* 1987;**125**:410–9.
30. Miracle-McMahill HL, Calle EE, Kosinski AS, Rodriguez C, Wingo PA, Thun MJ, et al. Tubal ligation and fatal ovarian cancer in a large prospective cohort study. *Am J Epidemiol.* 1997;**71**:948–51.

31. Greene A, Purdie D, Bain C, Siskind V, Russell P, Quinn M, et al. Tubal sterilisation, hysterectomy, and decreased risk of ovarian cancer. *Int J Cancer.* 1997;**145**:349–57.
32. Wingo P, Lee N, Ory H, Beral V, Peterson H, Rhodes P. Age-specific differences in the relationship between oral contraceptive use and breast cancer. *Cancer.* 1993;**71**:1506–17.
33. Winkler HA, Anderson PS, Fields AL, Runowicz CD, DeVictoria C, Goldberg GL. Compliance with Papanicolaou smear screening following tubal ligation in women with cervical cancer. *J Womens Health.* 1999;**8**:103–7.
34. Chi IC, Jones DB. Incidence, risk factors, and prevention of post-sterilisation regret in women: an updated review from an epidemiological prospective. *Obstet Gynaecol. Surv* 1994;**49**:722–32.
35. Glock JL, Kim AH, Hulka JF, Hunt RB, Trad FS, Brumsted JR. Reproductive outcome after tubal reversal in women 40 years of age or older. *Fertil Steril.* 1996;**65**:863–5.
36. Trimbos-Kemper TC. Reversal of sterilization in women over 40 years of age: a multicenter survey in The Netherlands. *Fertil Steril.* 1990;**53**:575–7.

INDEX